A DICTIONARY OF
EPIDEMIOLOGY

SECOND EDITION

Edited for the
International Epidemiological Association
by

John M. Last

New York   Oxford   Toronto
OXFORD UNIVERSITY PRESS
1988

Oxford University Press

Oxford   New York   Toronto
Delhi   Bombay   Calcutta   Madras   Karachi
Petaling Jaya   Singapore   Hong Kong   Tokyo
Nairobi   Dar es Salaam   Cape Town
Melbourne   Auckland

and associated companies in
Berlin   Ibadan

Library of Congress Cataloging-in-Publication Data

A Dictionary of epidemiology.
Includes bibliographies.
1. Epidemiology—Dictionaries.   I. Last, John M., 1926–   .
II. International Epidemiological Association.
[DNLM: 1. Epidemiology—dictionaries.
WA 13 D553]
RA651.D53   1988   614.4'03'21   87-31409
ISBN 0-19-505480-6
ISBN 0-19-505481-4 (pbk.)

2 4 6 8 10 9 7 5 3

Printed in the United States of America
on acid-free paper

Foreword

The International Epidemiological Association is extremely pleased that the *Dictionary of Epidemiology* has been so successful that a second edition has been demanded. As one of the Association's aims is to "spread the message," this work is an example of "what we call it." Only if we all understand the same thing when a particular term is used will the aim of the Association be capable of being fulfilled. This dictionary is fundamental to this objective.

W. W. Holland, MD FRCGP FRCP FFCM
President, International Epidemiological Association

Preface

This dictionary, appearing now in its second edition, is an attempt to bring some order to the occasionally chaotic nomenclature of epidemiology. It is intended for all who are interested in epidemiology, especially those who are beginning to study the subject, those whose first language is not English, and those from other fields who need to know the terms epidemiologists use.

Like all rapidly expanding sciences, epidemiology has been confounded by the proliferation of words and phrases to describe its concepts, principles, methods, and procedures. The creation of new terms and disagreement about the meaning of old ones can confuse beginners and established epidemiologists alike.

Remarks by users of the first edition have reinforced the view that the boundaries should be wide rather than narrow, that the language should be simple, that some terms many epidemiologists think everyone already knows should be included. The second edition is larger than the first, partly for this reason, and because terms omitted from the first edition have been included and many old entries expanded.

The dictionary is not an index of permitted and proscribed usage. I hope that it is authoritative without being authoritarian. Where synonyms exist, the definition appears under the most commonly used of these, but preference for one term over another is not necessarily implied. In a few instances, the use of a term is deprecated. Some terms that are properly described as slang or jargon have been included because they are widely used and their meaning is not always clear from the context. Murphy's description of jargon is worth recalling: "obscure and/or pretentious language, circumlocutions, invented meanings, and pomposity delighted in for its own sake."

There was disagreement among the contributors to this edition about including certain acronyms and eponyms. An acronym is a word made up of letters from two or more other words, e.g. ANOVA for analysis of variance, or from initial letters, e.g.

WHO for World Health Organization. All lay and technical vocabularies contain acronyms; epidemiology has its fair share. By convention, acronyms are spelt out the first time they appear in a text, and, if they are numerous, considerate editors sometimes supply a glossary, or at least list the acronyms along with the words for which they stand in an index. Although this dictionary is not the place for extensive mention of acronyms, a few appeared in the first edition, and a few more appear here.

Eponyms, the attachment of personal or place names to concepts, diseases, methods or specific studies, also occur often enough in published papers and books for us to recognize that beginners need some guidance to the meaning of those most widely used. Some appeared in the first edition, and a few have been added to the second—though again this dictionary is not the proper place for a full glossary of epidemiological eponyms (where would such a glossary end!).

As was the case with the first edition, a large number of epidemiologists from many countries have participated in this revision. The original modest notices in a couple of journals and a few casual remarks among friends produced a mailing list of some forty persons, mainly in North America and the United Kingdom. The mailing list rapidly grew until, by the fifth round of correspondence in December 1986, there were 108 correspondents in 25 countries. The list continued to grow after this fifth and final round; but the published roster of names that follows this preface is both more and less than the number of active participants. Some seemingly inquired just from curiosity and played no further part. Others wrote lengthy and often vigorously argumentative comments and suggestions expressing not only their own views but those of colleagues in their academic department or institution—in one instance, colleagues elsewhere in that nation.

In addition to extensive comments from these correspondents, I have made good use of other technical dictionaries and glossaries in compiling this revision. All of these are listed in the bibiliography, and many are also to be found in footnotes that follow specific entries.

The compilers of dictionaries must exercise the greatest care in the choice of words and in their arrangement. Most entries in this dictionary have been repeatedly discussed with many contributors, and in nearly all instances the wording has been agreed upon by all; on the rare occasions when agreement eluded us, the final decision was mine alone. Therefore, I accept full responsibility for the deficiencies in the finished product.

The work has been sponsored by the International Epidemiological Association, which provided partial travel support for me to attend two meetings in 1986; further support was provided by the McLean Foundation and the Milbank Memorial Fund. All royalties from the sale of this edition, like those from the first edition, will go to the International Epidemiological Association.

Finally, I thank Jeffrey House of Oxford University Press for helpful advice and encouragement.

Ottawa, Canada   J. M. L.
November 1987

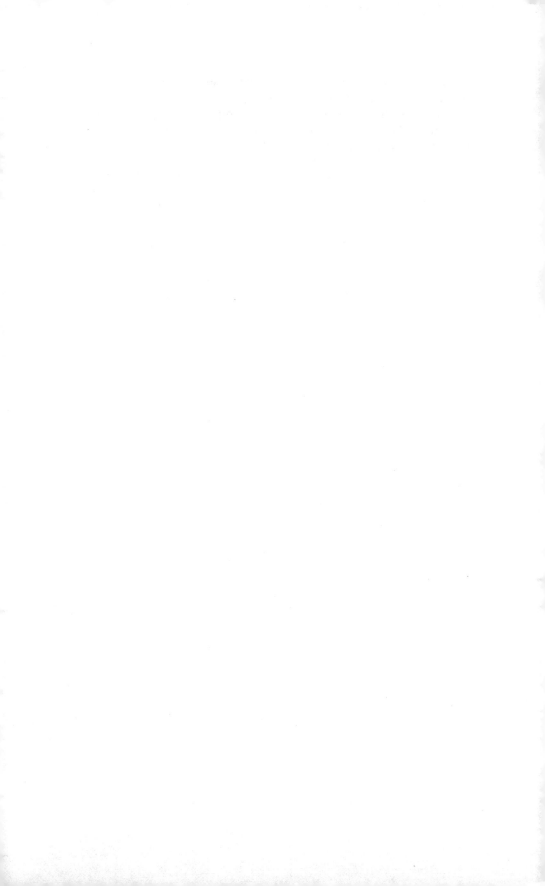

Contributing Editors

J. H. ABRAMSON
  Jerusalem, Israel

URSULA ACKERMAN-LIEBRICH
  Basel, Switzerland

ROBERT ALLARD
  Montreal, Quebec, Canada

JOHN C. BAILAR III
  Washington, DC, USA

CHRISTOPHER BALDOCK
  Brisbane, Queensland, Australia

ROBERTO G. BARUZZI
  São Paulo, Brazil

ABRAM S. BENENSON
  San Diego, CA, USA

ROGER BERNARD
  Geneva, Switzerland

JEAN-FRANÇOIS BOIVIN
  Montreal, Quebec, Canada

BERNARD J. BRABIN
  Madang, Papua New Guinea

C. RALPH BUNCHER
  Cincinnati, OH, USA

BEVERLEY CARLSON
  New York, NY, USA

JAMES CHIN
  Berkeley, CA, USA

MICHEL COLEMAN
  Oxford, England

L. CAYOLLA DA MOTTA
  Lisbon, Portugal

GARETH DAVIES
  New Haw, Surrey, England

RICHARD DICKER
  Atlanta, GA, USA

ALVAN R. FEINSTEIN
  New Haven, CT, USA

DAVID FINNEY
  Edinburgh, Scotland

JOSEPH L. FLEISS
  New York, NY, USA

GARY D. FRIEDMAN
  Oakland, CA, USA

MICHAEL GARRAWAY
  Edinburgh, Scotland

SANDER GREENLAND
  Los Angeles, CA, USA

TEE GUIDOTTI
  Edmonton, Alberta, Canada

WALTER W. HOLLAND
  London, England

BARBARA HULKA
  Chapel Hill, NC, USA

MICHEL IBRAHIM
  Chapel Hill, NC, USA

LESLIE M. IRWIG
  Sydney, NSW, Australia

MILOS JENICEK
  Montreal, Quebec, Canada

L. KARHAUSEN
  Luxembourg, Luxembourg

CORRESPONDING EDITORS

A Dictionary of Epidemiology

A

ABORTION RATE The estimated annual number of abortions per 1000 women of reproductive age (usually defined as age 15–44).

ABORTION RATIO The estimated number of abortions per 100 live births in a given year.

ABSCISSA The distance along the horizontal coordinate or x axis, of a point P from the vertical or y axis of a graph. See also AXIS, GRAPH, ORDINATE.

ABSOLUTE RISK Usually this term means the observed or calculated risk of an event in a population under study, as contrasted with the relative risk. Sometimes, however, it is a synonym for attributable fraction, excess risk, or risk difference; because of the inconsistency, this term should be avoided. See also RISK.

ACCEPTABLE RISK The risk that has minimal detrimental effects, or for which the benefits outweigh the potential hazards. Epidemiologic study has provided data for calculation of risks associated with many medical procedures and also with occupational and environmental exposures; these data are used, for instance, in CLINICAL DECISION ANALYSIS.

ACCURACY The degree to which a measurement, or an estimate based on measurements, represents the true value of the attribute that is being measured. See also MEASUREMENT, PROBLEMS WITH TERMINOLOGY.

ACQUAINTANCE NETWORK Group of persons in contact or communication among whom transmission of an infectious agent and of knowledge, attitudes, and values is possible, and whose social interaction may have health implications. See also TRANSMISSION OF INFECTION.

ACQUIRED IMMUNODEFICIENCY SYNDROME (Syn: acquired immune deficiency syndrome) (AIDS) For surveillance purposes, the Centers for Disease Control, Atlanta, Georgia,[1] define a case of AIDS as an illness characterized by (1) one or more of a group of opportunistic or indicator diseases that are indicative of underlying cellular immunodeficiency; (2) absence of all known underlying causes of cellular immunodeficiency and absence of all other causes of reduced resistance to opportunistic or indicator diseases. Additional criteria are serum positive for HIV antibody, positive culture for HIV, and reduction of T4 "helper" lymphocytes.

The opportunistic or indicator diseases associated with AIDS include certain protozoal and helminth infections, notably *Pneumocystis carinii* pneumonia and toxoplasmosis; fungal infections, notably candidiasis of esophagus, trachea, bronchi or lungs and cryptococcosis, especially affecting the central nervous system; bacterial infections, notably with certain mycobacteria; viral infections, notably cytomegalovirus and herpes simplex; and cancer, notably Kaposi's sarcoma and lymphoma limited to the brain.

AIDS-related complex (ARC) is the combination of HIV positive test with lymphadenopathy and persistent low fever but without immunodeficiency or opportunistic diseases.

[1] 1987 Revision of case definition of AIDS for surveillance purposes. MMWR 36, 1S:4S–9S, 1987.

ACTIVITIES OF DAILY LIVING (ADL) SCALE A scale devised by Katz and others[1] to score physical ability/disability; used to measure outcomes of interventions for various chronic disabling conditions such as arthritis. The scale is based on scores for responses to questions about mobility, self-care, grooming, etc. This was the first widely used scale of this type; others, mostly refinements or variations of the ADL scale, have since been developed.

[1] Katz S, Ford, AB, Moskowitz, RW, Jackson, BA, Jaffe, MW: Studies of illness in the aged. The index of ADL, a standardized measure of biological function. *JAMA* 185:914–919, 1963.

ACTUARIAL RATE See FORCE OF MORTALITY.

ACTUARIAL TABLE See LIFE TABLE.

ACUTE

1. Referring to a health effect, brief; sometimes loosely used to mean severe.
2. Referring to exposure, brief, intense, or short-term; sometimes specifically referring to brief exposure of high intensity. See also CHRONIC.

ADAPTATION A heritable component of the phenotype which confers an advantage in survival and reproductive success. The process by which organisms adapt to environmental conditions.

ADDITIVE MODEL A model in which the combined effect of several factors is the sum of the effects that would be produced by each of the factors in the absence of the others. For example, if factor X adds $x\%$ to risk in the absence of Y, and if factor Y adds $y\%$ to risk in the absence of X, an additive model states that the two factors together will add $(x+y)\%$ to risk. See also INTERACTION; LINEAR MODEL; MATHEMATICAL MODEL; MULTIPLICATIVE MODEL.

ADJUSTMENT A summarizing procedure for a statistical measure in which the effects of differences in composition of the populations being compared have been minimized by statistical methods. Examples are adjustment by regression analysis and by standardization. Adjustment often is performed on rates or relative risks, commonly because of differing age distributions in populations that are being compared. The mathematical procedure commonly used to adjust rates for age differences is direct or indirect standardization.

ADVERSE REACTION, SIDE EFFECT Any undesirable or unwanted consequence of a preventive, diagnostic, or therapeutic procedure.

AETIOLOGY, AETIOLOGIC See ETIOLOGY, ETIOLOGIC.

AGE DEPENDENCY RATIO See DEPENDENCY RATIO.

AGENT (OF DISEASE) A factor, such as a microorganism, chemical substance, or form of radiation, whose presence, excessive presence, or (in deficiency diseases) relative absence is essential for the occurrence of a disease. A disease may have a single agent, a number of independent alternative agents (at least one of which must be present), or a complex of two or more factors whose combined presence is essential for the development of the disease. See also CAUSALITY; NECESSARY AND SUFFICIENT CAUSE.

AGE–PERIOD COHORT ANALYSIS See COHORT ANALYSIS.

AGE–SEX PYRAMID See POPULATION PYRAMID.

AGE–SEX REGISTER List of all clients or patients of a medical practice or service, classified by age (birthdate) and sex; provides denominator for calculating age- and sex-specific rates.

AGE-SPECIFIC FERTILITY RATE The number of births occurring during a specified period to women of a specified age group, divided by the number of person-years lived during that period by women of that age group. When an age-specific fertility rate is calculated for a calendar year, the number of births to women of the specified age is usually divided by the midyear population of women of that age.

AGE-SPECIFIC RATE A rate for a specified age group. The numerator and denominator refer to the same age group.

Example:

$$\text{Age-specific death rate (age 25–34)} = \frac{\text{Number of deaths among residents age 25–34 in an area in a year}}{\text{Average (or midyear) population age 25–34 in the area in that year}} \times 100,000$$

The multiplier (usually 100,000 or 1,000,000) is chosen to produce a rate that can be expressed as a convenient number.

AGE STANDARDIZATION A procedure for adjusting rates, e.g. death rates, designed to minimize the effects of differences in age composition when comparing rates for different populations. See also ADJUSTMENT, STANDARDIZATION.

AGGREGATION BIAS (Syn: ecological bias) See ECOLOGICAL FALLACY.

AGING OF THE POPULATION A demographic term, meaning an increase over time in the proportion of older persons in the population. It does not necessarily imply an increase in life expectancy or that "people are living longer than they used to." The principal determinant of aging in the population has been a decline in the birth rate: when fewer children are born than in prior years, the result, in the absence of a rise in the death rate at higher ages, has been an increase in the proportion of older persons in the population. In developed societies, however, mortality change is becoming a factor: little further mortality reduction can occur in the first half of life, so reductions are beginning to occur in the third and fourth quarters of life, leading to a rise in the proportion of older persons from this cause.

AIRBORNE INFECTION A mechanism of transmission of an infectious agent by particles, dust, or DROPLET NUCLEI suspended in the air. See also TRANSMISSION OF INFECTION.

ALGORITHM Any systematic process that consists of an ordered sequence of steps with each step depending on the outcome of the previous one. The term is commonly used to describe a structured process, for instance, relating to computer programming or to health planning. See also DECISION TREE.

ALGORITHM, CLINICAL (Syn: clinical protocol) An explicit description of steps to be taken in patient care in specified circumstances. This approach makes use of branching logic and of all pertinent data, both about the patient and from epidemiologic and other sources, to arrive at decisions that yield maximum benefit and minimum risk.

ALLELE Alternative forms of a gene, occupying the same locus on a chromosome.

ALPHA ERROR See ERROR, TYPE I.

ALPHA LEVEL See SIGNIFICANCE LEVEL.

ANALYSIS OF VARIANCE A statistical technique that isolates and assesses the contribution of categorical independent variables to variation in the mean of a continuous dependent variable. The observations are classified according to their categories for each of the independent variables, and the differences between the categories in their mean values on the dependent variable are estimated and tested for statistical significance.

ANALYTIC STUDY A study designed to examine associations, commonly putative or hypothesized causal relationships. An analytic study is usually concerned with identifying or measuring the effects of risk factors, or is concerned with the health effects of specific exposure(s). Contrast descriptive study, which does not test hypotheses. The common types of analytic study are CROSS-SECTIONAL, COHORT, and CASE-CONTROL. In an analytic study, individuals in the study population may be classified according to absence or presence (or future development) of specific disease and according to "attributes" that may influence disease occurrence. Attributes may include age, race, sex, other disease(s), genetic, biochemical, and physiological characteristics, economic status, occupation, residence, and various aspects of the environment or personal behavior. See also CASE CONTROL STUDY; COHORT STUDY; CROSS-SECTIONAL STUDY; STUDY DESIGN.

ANIMAL MODEL Study in a population of laboratory animals that uses conditions of animals analogous to conditions of humans to model processes comparable to those that occur in human populations. See also EXPERIMENTAL EPIDEMIOLOGY.

ANTAGONISM Opposite of SYNERGISM. The situation in which the combined effect of two or more factors is smaller than the solitary effect of any one of the factors. In BIOASSAY, the term may be used to refer to the situation when a specified response is produced by exposure to either of two factors but not by exposure to both together.

ANTHROPOMETRY The technique that deals with the measurement of the size, weight, and proportions of the human body.

ANTHROPOPHILIC (adj.) Pertaining to an insect's preference for feeding on humans even when nonhuman hosts are available.

ANTIBODY Protein molecule formed by exposure to a "foreign" or extraneous substance, e.g., invading microorganisms responsible for infection, or active immunization. May also be present as a result of passive transfer from mother to infant, via immune globulin, etc. Antibody has the capacity to bind specifically to the foreign substance (antigen) that elicited its production, thus supplying a mechanism for protection against infectious diseases. Antibody is epidemiologically important because its concentration (titer) can be measured in individuals, and, therefore, in populations. See also SEROEPIDEMIOLOGY.

ANTIGEN A substance (protein, polysaccharide, glycolipid, tissue transplant, etc.) that is capable of inducing specific immune response. Introduction of antigen may be by the invasion of infectious organisms, immunization, inhalation, ingestion, etc.

ANTIGENIC DRIFT This term describes the "evolutionary" changes that take place in the molecular structure of DNA/RNA in micro-organisms during their passage from one host to another. It may be due to recombination, deletion or insertion of genes, to point mutations, or to several of these events. This process has been studied in common viruses, notably the influenza virus.[1] It leads to alteration (usually slow and progressive) in the antigenic composition, and thus in the immunologic responses of individuals and populations to exposure to the micro-organisms concerned. See also ANTIGENIC SHIFT.

[1] Palese P, Young JF: Variation of Influenza A, B, and C Viruses. *Science* 215:1468–1473, 1982.

ANTIGENIC SHIFT This term describes mutation, i.e., a sudden change in molecular structure of DNA/RNA in micro-organisms, especially viruses, which produces new strains of the micro-organism. Hosts previously exposed to other strains have little or no acquired immunity. Antigenic shift is believed to be the explanation for the occurrence of strains of the influenza A virus associated with large-scale epidemic and pandemic spread. Antigenic shift is responsible for the susceptibility of host populations to a new strain of influenza virus. See also ANTIGENIC DRIFT.

ANTIGENICITY (Syn: immunogenicity) The ability of agent(s) to produce a systemic or a local immunologic reaction in the host.

ARBOVIRUS A group of taxonomically diverse animal viruses that are unified by an epidemiologic concept, i.e., transmission between vertebrate host organisms by blood-feeding (hematophagous) arthropod vectors such as mosquitoes, ticks, sand flies, and midges. The term is a contraction of *arthropod-borne virus*.

The interaction of arbovirus, vertebrate host(s), and arthropod vector gives this class of infections several unique epidemiologic features. See VECTOR-BORNE INFECTION for definition of terms used to describe these features.

AREA SAMPLING A method of sampling that can be used when the numbers in the population are unknown. The total area to be sampled is divided into subareas, e.g., by means of a grid that produces squares on a map; these subareas are then numbered and sampled, using a table of random numbers. Depending upon circumstances, the population in the sampled areas may first be enumerated, then a second stage of sampling may be conducted.

ARITHMETIC MEAN The sum of all the values in a set of measurements, divided by the number of values in the set.

ARTIFICIAL INTELLIGENCE A branch of computer science in which attempts are made to duplicate human intellectual functions. One application is in diagnosis, in which computer programs are often based upon epidemiologic analyses of data in hospital charts or other clinical records.

ASCERTAINMENT The process of determining what is happening in a population or study group, e.g., family and household composition, occurrence of cases of specific diseases; the latter is also known as case-finding.

ASCERTAINMENT BIAS Systematic failure to represent equally all classes of cases or persons supposed to be represented in a sample. This bias may arise because of the nature of the sources from which persons come, e.g., a specialized clinic; from a diagnostic process influenced by culture, custom, or idiosyncracy; or, for example, in genetic studies, from the statistical chance of selecting from large or small families.

ASSAY The quantitative or qualitative evaluation of a hazardous substance; the results of such an evaluation.

ASSOCIATION (Syn: correlation, [statistical] dependence, relationship) Statistical dependence between two or more events, characteristics, or other variables. An association is present if the probability of occurrence of an event or characteristic, or the quantity of a variable, depends upon the occurrence of one or more other events, the presence of one or more other characteristics, or the quantity of one or more other variables. The association between two variables is described as positive when the occurrence of higher values of a variable is associated with the occurrence of higher values of another variable. In a negative association, the occurrence of higher values of one variable is associated with lower values of the other variable. An association may be fortuitous or may be produced by various other circumstances; the presence of an association does not necessarily imply a causal relationship. If the use of the term "association" is confined to situations in which the relationship between two variables is statistically significant, the terms "statistical association" and "statistically significant association" become tautological. However, ordinary usage is seldom so precise as this. The terms "association" and "relationship" are often used interchangeably.

Associations can be broadly grouped under two headings, symmetrical or noncausal (see below) and asymmetrical or causal.

ASSOCIATION, ASYMMETRICAL (Syn: asymmetrical relationship) The definitive conditions of asymmetrical associations are direction and time. Independent variable X must cause changes in dependent variable $Y,$ and the "causal" variable must precede its "effects." Bradford Hill[1] and others[2,3] have pointed out that the (subjective) likelihood of a causal relationship is increased by the presence of the following attributes. However, temporality is the only indispensable condition among these.

1. Consistency—The association is consistent if the results are replicated when studied in different settings and by different methods.
2. Strength—This is an expression of the disparity between the frequency with which a factor is found in the disease and the frequency with which it occurs in the absence of the disease. Not to be confused with statistical significance.
3. Specificity—This is established with the limitation of the association to a single putative cause and single effect.
4. Dose–response relationship—This is established when an increased risk or severity in disease occurs with an increased quantity ("dose") or duration of exposure to a factor.
5. Temporality—The exposure to a putative cause always precedes, never follows, the outcome.
6. Biological plausibility—It is desirable that the association agree with current understanding of the response of cells, tissues, organs, and systems to stimuli. This criterion should not be applied rigidly. The association may be new to science or medicine. As Sherlock Holmes advised Dr. Watson, "When you have eliminated the impossible, whatever remains, however improbable, must be the truth."
7. Coherence—The associations should not *conflict* with the generally known facts of the natural history and biology of disease.
8. Experiment—It is sometimes possible to appeal to experimental, or quasi-experimental evidence, e.g., an observed association leads to some preventive action. Does this action in fact prevent?

See also CAUSALITY: EVANS'S POSTULATES; KOCH'S POSTULATES.

[1] Bradford Hill A: The environment and disease: Association or causation. *Proc Roy Soc Med* 58:295–300, 1965.
[2] Susser MW: Judgment and causal inference. *Am J Epidemiol* 105:1–15, 1977.
[3] Rothman KJ (Ed): *Causal Inference.* Chestnut Hill, MA: Epidemiology Resources Inc., 1988.

ASSOCIATION, DIRECT Directly associated, i.e., not via a known third variable: $A \rightarrow B$. Refers only to causality.

ASSOCIATION, INDIRECT CAUSAL Two types are distinguished:

1. Association of a factor C with disease A only because both are related to a common underlying factor B.

$$A \overset{B}{\underset{\nwarrow \; \searrow}{}} C$$

Alteration of factor C will not produce an alteration in the frequency to disease A unless an alteration in C affects B. It has been suggested that to avoid confusion with the alternative meaning of *indirect association*, this type should be called "secondary association."

2. Association of a factor C with disease A by means of an intermediate or intervening factor B.

$$C \overset{B}{\underset{\nearrow \; \searrow}{}} A$$

Alteration of factor C would produce an alteration in the frequency of disease A. To avoid confusion, this type should be called "indirect causal association."

ASSOCIATION, SPURIOUS A term, preferably avoided, used with different meanings by different authors. It may refer to artifactual, fortuitous, false secondary, or to all kinds of noncausal associations due to chance, bias, failure to control for extraneous variables, etc.

ASSOCIATION, SYMMETRICAL An association is noncausal if it is symmetrical, as in the statement $F = MA$ (force equals mass times acceleration). This is a noncausal, non-directional expression of the mathematical relationship between the physical properties of force, mass, and velocity. If one side of the equation is changed, then the other must also change to maintain equilibrium.

Although epidemiologists are usually most interested in asymmetrical statements that have direction, the symmetrical equation can be useful. For instance, prevalence can be expressed in terms of incidence and duration in the simple equation, $P = I \times D$. If two of these three elements are known, the third can be derived. See also SYMMETRICAL RELATIONSHIP.

ASSORTATIVE MATING Selection of a mate with preference (or aversion) for a particular genotype, i.e., nonrandom mating.

ASYMMETRICAL ASSOCIATION See ASSOCIATION, ASYMMETRICAL.

ASYMPTOTIC Pertaining to a limiting value, for example, of a dependent variable, when the independent variable approaches zero or infinity. See LARGE SAMPLE METHOD.

ASYMPTOTIC METHOD See LARGE SAMPLE METHOD.

ATTACK RATE Attack rate, or case rate, is a CUMULATIVE INCIDENCE RATE often used for particular groups, observed for limited periods and under special circumstances, as in an epidemic.

The *secondary attack rate* is the number of cases among contacts occurring within the accepted incubation period following exposure to a primary case, in relation to the total of exposed contacts; the denominator may be restricted to susceptible contacts when determinable.

Infection rate is the incidence of manifest plus inapparent infections, which can be identified, e.g., by SEROEPIDEMIOLOGY.

ATTRIBUTABLE FRACTION (AF) (Syn: attributable proportion) A term sometimes used to refer to the attributable fraction in the population, and sometimes to the attributable fraction among the exposed. See also ATTRIBUTABLE FRACTION (EXPOSED); ATTRIBUTABLE FRACTION (POPULATION).

ATTRIBUTABLE FRACTION (EXPOSED) (Syn: attributable proportion [exposed], attributable risk, etiologic fraction [exposed]). With a given outcome, exposure factor and population, the attributable fraction among the exposed is the proportion by which the incidence rate of the outcome among those exposed would be reduced if the exposure were eliminated. It may be estimated by the formula

$$AF_e = \frac{I_e - I_u}{I_e}$$

where I_e is the incidence rate among the exposed, I_u is the incidence rate among the unexposed; or by the formula

$$AF_e = \frac{RR - 1}{RR}$$

where RR is the rate ratio, I_e/I_u. It is assumed that causes other than the one under investigation have had equal effects on the exposed and unexposed groups.

ATTRIBUTABLE FRACTION (POPULATION) (Syn: attributable proportion [population], etiologic fraction [population], attributable risk). With a given outcome, exposure factor, and population, the attributable fraction among the population is the proportion by which the incidence rate of the outcome in the entire population would be reduced if exposure were eliminated. It may be estimated by the formula

$$AF_{\mathrm{p}} = \frac{I_{\mathrm{p}} - I_{\mathrm{u}}}{I_{\mathrm{p}}}$$

where I_{p} is the incidence rate in the total population and I_{u} is the incidence rate among the unexposed; or by the formula

$$\frac{P_{\mathrm{e}}(RR - 1)}{1 + P_{\mathrm{e}}(RR - 1)}$$

where RR is the rate ratio, $I_{\mathrm{u}}/I_{\mathrm{p}}$. It is assumed that causes other than the one under investigation have had equal effects on the exposed and unexposed groups.

ATTRIBUTABLE NUMBER The number of new occurrences of a specific outcome attributable to an exposure; it may be estimated using the formula

$$AN = \frac{I_{\mathrm{e}} - I_{\mathrm{u}}}{N_{\mathrm{e}}}$$

where I_{e} is the incidence rate among the exposed, I_{u} is the incidence rate among the unexposed, and N_{e} is the number of persons in the exposed population. It is assumed that causes other than the one under investigation have had equal effects on the exposed and unexposed groups.

ATTRIBUTABLE RISK The rate of a disease or other outcome in exposed individuals that can be attributed to the exposure. This measure is derived by subtracting the rate of the outcome (usually incidence or mortality) among the unexposed from the rate among the exposed individuals; it is assumed that causes other than the one under investigation have had equal effects on the exposed and unexposed groups. Unfortunately, this term has been used to denote a number of different concepts, including the attributable fraction in the population, the attributable fraction among the exposed, the population excess rate, and the rate difference. Therefore, it should be defined carefully by all who use it. See also ATTRIBUTABLE FRACTION (EXPOSED); POPULATION EXCESS RATE; ATTRIBUTABLE FRACTION (POPULATION); POPULATION ATTRIBUTABLE RISK; RATE DIFFERENCE.

ATTRIBUTABLE RISK (EXPOSED) This term has been used with different connotations to denote the attributable fraction among the exposed and the excess risk among the exposed. See also ATTRIBUTABLE FRACTION (EXPOSED); RATE DIFFERENCE.

ATTRIBUTABLE RISK (POPULATION) This term has been used with different connotations to denote the attributable fraction in the population and the population excess risk. See also ATTRIBUTABLE FRACTION (POPULATION); POPULATION EXCESS RATE.

ATTRIBUTABLE RISK PERCENT Attributable fraction expressed as a percentage rather than as a proportion.

ATTRIBUTABLE RISK PERCENT (EXPOSED) This is the attributable fraction among the exposed, expressed as a percentage. See also ATTRIBUTABLE FRACTION (EXPOSED).

ATTRIBUTABLE RISK PERCENT (POPULATION) This is the attributable fraction in the population, expressed as a percentage. See also ATTRIBUTABLE FRACTION (POPULATION).

ATTRIBUTE A qualitative characteristic of an individual or item.

AUDIT An examination or review that establishes the extent to which a condition, process, or performance conforms to predetermined standards or criteria.

AUTOPSY DATA Data derived from autopsied deaths, e.g., for study of natural history of disease and trends in frequency of disease. Autopsies are done on nonrandomly selected persons in the population and findings should therefore be generalized only with great caution.

AVERAGE Kendall and Buckland's *Dictionary of Statistical Terms* (4th Edition, 1982) has this to say: "A familiar but elusive concept. Generally an 'average' value purports to represent or to summarize the relevant features of a set of values; and in this sense the term would include the median and the mode. In a more limited sense an 'average' compounds all the values of the set, e.g., in the case of the arithmetic or geometric means. In ordinary usage, 'the average' is often understood to refer to the arithmetic mean." See also MEASURES OF CENTRAL TENDENCY.

AVERAGE LIFE EXPECTANCY See EXPECTATION OF LIFE.

AXIS

1. One of the dimensions of a graph. A two-dimensional graph has two axes, the horizontal or x axis, and the vertical or y axis. Mathematically, there may be more than two axes, and graphs are sometimes drawn with a third dimension; the eye cannot comprehend more than three dimensions.

2. In NOSOLOGY, an axis of classification is the conceptual framework, e.g., etiologic, topographic, psychologic, sociologic. The International Classification of Disease, for example, is multiaxial; the primary axis is topographic (i.e., body systems); secondary axes relate to etiology, manifestations of disease, detail of sites affected, severity, etc.

B

BACKGROUND LEVEL, RATE The concentration, often low, at which some substance, agent, or event is present or occurs at a particular time and place in the absence of a specific hazard or set of hazards under investigation. An example is the background level of naturally occurring forms of ionizing radiation to which we are all exposed.

BAR DIAGRAM A graphic technique for presenting DISCRETE DATA organized in such a way that each observation can fall into one and only one category of the variable. Frequencies are listed along one axis and categories of the variable along the other axis. The frequencies of each group of observations are represented by the lengths of the corresponding bars. See also HISTOGRAM.

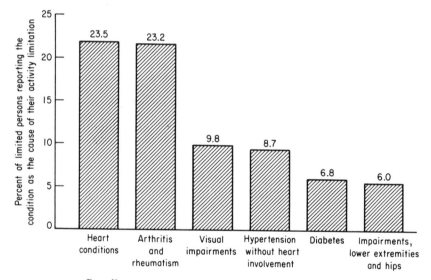

Bar diagram. *From* Susser, Watson, Hopper, 1985.

BAYES' THEOREM A theorem in probability theory named for Thomas Bayes (1702–1761), an English clergyman and mathematician; his *Essay Towards Solving a Problem in the Doctrine of Chances* (1763, published posthumously), contained this theorem. In epidemiology, it is used to obtain the probability of disease in a group of people with some characteristic on the basis of the overall rate of that disease (the prior probability of disease) and of the likelihoods of that characteristic in healthy and diseased individuals. The most familiar application is in CLINICAL DECISION ANALYSIS where it is used for estimating the probability of a particular diagnosis given the appearance of some symptoms or test result. A simplified version of the theorem is

$$P(D|S) = \frac{P(S|D)P(D)}{P(S|D)P(D) + P(S|\overline{D})P(\overline{D})}$$

where D = disease, S = symptom, and $\overline{D}$ = no disease. The formula emphasizes what clinical intuition often overlooks, namely, that the probability of disease given this symptom depends not only on how characteristic that symptom is of the disease but also on how frequent the disease is among the population being served. "If you hear hoof beats in the street, do not look for zebra."

The theorem can also be used for estimating exposure-specific rates from case control studies if there is added information about the overall rate of disease in that population.

Some of the terms in the theorem have special names. The probability of disease given the symptom is called the "posterior probability." It is an estimate of the probability of disease posterior to knowing whether or not the symptom was present. The overall probability of disease among the population or our guess of the probability of disease before knowing of the presence or absence of the symptom is called the "prior probability." The theorem is sometimes presented in terms of the odds of disease before knowing the symptom (prior odds) and after knowing the symptom (posterior odds).

BEHAVIORAL EPIDEMIC An epidemic originating in behavioral patterns (as opposed to invading microorganisms or physical agents). Examples include the dancing manias of the Middle Ages, episodes of mass fainting or convulsions ("hysterical epidemics"), crowd panic, or waves of fashion or enthusiasm. The communicable nature of the behavior is dependent not only on person-to-person transmission of the behavioral pattern but also on group reinforcement (as with smoking, alcohol, or drug use). Behavioral epidemics may be difficult to differentiate from, or may complicate, outbreaks of organic disease, for example, due to contamination of the environment by a toxic substance.

BEHAVIORAL RISK FACTOR A characteristic or behavior that is associated with increased probability of a specified outcome; the term does not imply a causal relationship.

BENCHMARK A slang or jargon term, usually meaning a measurement taken at the outset of a series of measurements of the same variable, sometimes meaning the best or most desirable value of the variable. Because of uncertainty about meaning, the term should not be used.

BENEFIT–COST RATIO The ratio of net present value of measurable benefits to costs. Calculation of a benefit–cost ratio is used to determine the economic feasibility or success of a program.

BERNOULLI DISTRIBUTION The probability distribution associated with two mutually exclusive and exhaustive outcomes, e.g., death or survival; a Bernoulli variable is one that has only two possible values, e.g., death or survival. See also BINOMIAL DISTRIBUTION.

BERKSON'S BIAS See BIAS, SELECTION.

BETA ERROR See ERROR, TYPE II.

BIAS Deviation of results or inferences from the truth, or processes leading to such deviation. Any trend in the collection, analysis, interpretation, publication, or review of data that can lead to conclusions that are systematically different from the truth. Among the ways in which deviation from the truth can occur, are the following:

1. Systematic (one-sided) variation of measurements from the true values (syn: systematic error).

2. Variation of statistical summary measures (means, rates, measures of association, etc.) from their true values as a result of systematic variation of measurements, other flaws in data collection, or flaws in study design or analysis.
3. Deviation of inferences from the truth as a result of flaws in study design, data collection, or the analysis or interpretation of results.
4. A tendency of procedures (in study design, data collection, analysis, interpretation, review or publication) to yield results or conclusions that depart from the truth.
5. Prejudice leading to the conscious or unconscious selection of study procedures that depart from the truth in a particular direction, or to one-sidedness in the interpretation of results.

The term "bias" does not necessarily carry an imputation of prejudice or other subjective factor, such as the experimenter's desire for a particular outcome. This differs from conventional usage in which bias refers to a partisan point of view.

Many varieties of bias have been described.[1]

[1] Sackett DL: Bias in analytic research. *J Chron Dis* 32:51–63, 1979.

BIAS, ASCERTAINMENT Systematic error, arising from the kind of individuals or patients (e.g., slightly ill, moderately ill, acutely ill) that the individual observer is seeing. Also systematic error arising from the diagnostic process (which may be determined by the culture, customs, or individual idiosyncrasy of the person providing care for the patient).

BIAS, IN ASSUMPTION (Syn: conceptual bias) Error arising from faulty logic or premises or mistaken beliefs on the part of the investigator. False conclusions about the explanation for associations between variables. Example: Having correctly deduced the mode of transmission of cholera, John Snow concluded that yellow fever was transmitted by similar means. In fact, the "miasma" theory would better fit the facts of yellow fever transmission.

BIAS IN AUTOPSY SERIES Systematic error resulting from the fact that autopsies represent a nonrandom sample of all deaths.

BIAS, BERKSON'S See BIAS, SELECTION.

BIAS DUE TO CONFOUNDING See CONFOUNDING.

BIAS, DESIGN The difference between a true value and that actually obtained, occurring as a result of faulty design of a study. Some examples are (1) uncontrolled studies where the effects of two processes cannot be separated (confounding), (2) controlled studies where observations are based on a poorly defined population, and (3) nonsimultaneous comparisons, e.g., use of historical controls.

BIAS, DETECTION Due to systematic error(s) in methods of ascertainment, diagnosis, or verification of cases in an epidemiologic survey, study, or investigation. Example: Verification of diagnosis by laboratory tests in hospital cases, but failure to apply the same tests to cases outside the hospital.

BIAS DUE TO DIGIT PREFERENCE See DIGIT PREFERENCE.

BIAS IN HANDLING OUTLIERS Error arising from a failure to discard an unusual value occurring in a small sample, or due to exclusion of unusual values that should be included.

BIAS, INFORMATION (Syn: observational bias) A flaw in measuring exposure or outcome that results in differential quality (accuracy) of information between compared groups.

BIAS DUE TO INSTRUMENTAL ERROR Systematic error due to faulty calibration, inaccurate measuring instruments, contaminated reagents, incorrect dilution or mixing of reagents, etc.

BIAS OF INTERPRETATION Error arising from inference and speculation. Sources of the error include (1) failure of the investigator to consider every interpretation consistent with the facts and to assess the credentials of each, and (2) mishandling of cases that constitute exceptions to some general conclusion.

BIAS, INTERVIEWER Systematic error due to interviewers' subconscious or even conscious gathering of selective data.

BIAS, "LEAD-TIME" A systematic error arising when follow-up of two groups does not begin at strictly comparable times. Occurs especially when one group has been diagnosed earlier in the natural history of the disease than the other group. See also ZERO TIME SHIFT.

BIAS, LENGTH A systematic error due to the selection of a disproportionate number of long-duration cases (cases who survive longest) in one group and not in the other. Can occur when prevalent cases, rather than incident cases, are included in a case control study.

BIAS, MEASUREMENT Systematic error arising from inaccurate measurement (or classification) of subjects on the study variables.

BIAS, OBSERVER Systematic difference between a true value and that actually observed due to observer variation. Observer variation may be due to differences among observers (interobserver variation) or to variation in readings by the same observer on separate occasions (intraobserver variation). See also OBSERVER VARIATION.

BIAS IN THE PRESENTATION OF DATA Error due to irregularities produced by DIGIT PREFERENCE, incomplete data, poor techniques of measurement, or technically poor laboratory standards.

BIAS IN PUBLICATION An editorial predilection for publishing particular findings, e.g., positive results, which leads to the failure of authors to submit negative findings for publication or failure of journal editors to accept and publish reports with negative findings. This can distort the general belief about what has been demonstrated in a particular situation.

BIAS OF AN ESTIMATOR The difference between the expected value of an estimator of a parameter and the true value of this parameter. See also UNBIASSED ESTIMATOR.

BIAS, RECALL Systematic error due to differences in accuracy or completeness of recall to memory of prior events or experiences. Example: Mothers whose children have had or have died of leukemia are more likely than mothers of healthy living children to remember details of diagnostic x-ray examinations to which these children were exposed in utero.

BIAS, REPORTING Selective suppression or revealing of information such as past history of sexually transmitted disease.

BIAS, RESPONSE Systematic error due to difference in characteristics between those who choose or volunteer to participate in a study and those who do not.

BIAS, SAMPLING Unless the sampling method ensures that all members of the "universe" or reference population have a known chance of selection in the sample, bias is possible. The best way to ensure a known chance of selection for all is to use a probability sampling method such as a table of random numbers.

BIAS, SELECTION Error due to systematic differences in characteristics between those who are selected for study and those who are not. Examples include hospital cases or cases under a physician's care, excluding those who die before admission to hospital because the course of their disease is so acute, those not sick enough to require hospital care, or those excluded by distance, cost, or other factors. Selection bias also invalidates generalizable conclusions from surveys that would include only volunteers from a healthy population.

A special example is BERKSON'S BIAS,[1] which Berkson characterized as the set of selective factors that lead hospital cases and controls in a case control study to be systematically different from one another. This occurs when the combination of exposure and disease under study increases the risk of hospital admission, thus leading to a systematically higher exposure rate among the hospital cases than the hospital controls. This in turn results in systematic distortion of the ODDS RATIO.

[1] Berkson J: Limitations of the application of fourfold table analysis to hospital data. *Biometrics Bull* 2:47–53, 1946.

BIAS DUE TO WITHDRAWALS A difference between the true value and that actually observed in a study due to the characteristics of those subjects who choose to withdraw.

BILLS OF MORTALITY Weekly and annual abstracts of christenings and burials, distinguishing deaths from the plague, compiled for London (and some other cities), especially in times of plague, from the English parish registers that started in 1538. From 1629, the annual bill was published regularly and included a breakdown of deaths by cause. These records were the basis for the earliest vital statistics, compiled, analyzed, and discussed by John Graunt in *Natural and Political Observations . . . on the Bills of Mortality* (1662).

BIMODAL DISTRIBUTION A distribution with two regions of high frequency separated by a region of low frequency of observations. A two-peak distribution.

BINARY VARIABLE A variable having only two possible values, e.g. on or off, 0 or 1. See also BIT.

BINOMIAL DISTRIBUTION A probability distribution associated with two mutually exclusive outcomes, e.g., presence or absence of a clinical or laboratory sign, death, or survival. The probability distribution of the number of occurrences of a binary event in a sample of n independent observations. The binomial distribution is used to model CUMULATIVE INCIDENCE RATES and PREVALENCE RATES. The BERNOULLI DISTRIBUTION is a special case of the binomial distribution with $n = 1$.

BIOASSAY The quantitative evaluation of the potency of a substance by assessing its effects on tissues, cells, live experimental animals, or humans.

Bioassay may be a direct method of estimating relative potency: groups of subjects are assigned to each of two (or more) preparations; the dose that is just sufficient to produce a specified response is measured, and the estimate is the ratio of the mean doses for the two (or more) groups. In this method, the death of the subject may be used as the "response."

The indirect method (more commonly used) requires study of the relationship between the magnitude of a dose and the magnitude of a quantitative response produced by it.

BIOLOGICAL PLAUSIBILITY The criterion that an observed, presumably or putatively causal ASSOCIATION fits previously existing biological or medical knowledge. This judgment should be used cautiously since it could impede development of new knowledge that does not fit existing ideas.

BIOLOGICAL TRANSMISSION See VECTOR-BORNE INFECTION.

BIOMETRY [literally, the *measurement of life*] The application of statistical methods to the study of numerical data based on biological observations and phenomena. The term was coined by W. F. R. Weldon (1860–1906), a zoologist at University College, London. FRANCIS GALTON has been called "the father of biometry" for his application of statistical methods to the analysis of biological variation. However, others preceded him, e.g., QUETELET and LOUIS.

BIOSTATISTICS Application of STATISTICS to biological problems. The term is considered by many biomedical scientists to mean the application of statistics specifically to medical problems, but its real meaning is broader.

BIRAUD, YVES (1900–1965) French physician and statistician. He served the League of Nations and later WHO as Director of Epidemiological and Statistical Services from 1925 to 1960. In 1960, he founded the first chair of Health Statistics in France, at the *Ecole de santé publique* in Rennes.

BIRTH CERTIFICATE Official, legal document recording details of a live birth, usually comprising name, date, place, identity of parents, and sometimes additional information such as birth weight. It provides the basis for vital statistics of birth and birthrates in a political or administrative jurisdiction, and for the denominator for infant mortality and certain other vital rates.

BIRTH COHORT See COHORT.

BIRTH COHORT ANALYSIS See COHORT ANALYSIS.

BIRTH INTERVAL Interval between termination of one completed pregnancy and the termination of the next.

BIRTH ORDER The ranking of siblings according to age, starting with the eldest in a family. The ordinal number of a given live birth in relation to all previous live births of the same women. Thus, 4 is the birth order of the fourth live birth occurring to the same woman. This strict demographic definition may be loosened to include all births, i.e., still-births as well as live births

BIRTH RATE A summary rate based on the number of live births in a population over a given period, usually one year.

$$\text{Birth rate} = \frac{\text{Number of live births to residents in an area in a calendar year}}{\text{Average or midyear population in the area in that year}} \times 1000$$

BIRTH WEIGHT Infant's weight recorded at the time of birth and, in some countries, entered on the birth certificate. Certain variants of birth weight are precisely defined. Low birth weight (LBW) is below 2500 g. Very low birth weight (VLBW) is below 1500 g. Ultralow birth weight (ULBW) is below 1000 g. Large for gestational age (LGA) is birth weight above the 90th percentile. Average weight for gestational age (AGA) (Syn: appropriate or adequate): birth weight between 10th and 90th percentiles. Small for gestational age (SGA) (Syn: small for dates): birth weight below 10th percentile.

BIT Acronym for binary digit; the signal in computing. See also BYTE.

"BLACK BOX" A jargon term, meaning a method of reasoning or studying a problem, in which the methods, procedures, etc., as such are not described, explained, or perhaps even understood. Nothing is stated or inferred about the method; discussion and conclusions relate solely to the empirical relationships observed. An alternative definition is the following: A method of formally relating an input, e.g., quantity of a drug absorbed over a period or a putative causal factor, to an output, e.g., the amount of the drug eliminated in a given period, or an observed effect, without making detailed assumptions about the mechanisms that have contributed to the transformation of input to output within the organism (the "black box").

BLIND(ED) STUDY (Syn: masked study) A study in which observer(s) and/or subjects are kept ignorant of the group to which the subjects are assigned, as in an experiment, or of the population from which the subjects come, as in a nonexperimental study. When both observer and subjects are kept ignorant, we refer to a double-blind study. If the statistical analysis is also done in ignorance of the group to which subjects belong, the study is sometimes described as triple-blind. The intent of keeping subjects and/or investigators blinded, i.e., unaware of knowledge that might introduce a bias, is to eliminate the effects of such biases. To avoid confusion about the meaning of the word "blind" some authors prefer to describe such studies as "masked."

BLOCKED RANDOMIZATION See STRATIFIED RANDOMIZATION. The analogue in a randomized experiment of individual matching in an observational study.

BODY MASS INDEX (Syn: Quetelet's index) One of the anthropometric measures of body mass. Defined as (weight) $\div$ (height)^2. This measure has the highest correlation with skinfold thickness or body density and in this respect is superior to the PONDERAL INDEX.

BOOTSTRAP A technique for estimating the variance and the bias of an estimator by repeatedly drawing random samples with replacement from the observations at hand. One applies the estimator to each sample drawn, thus obtaining a set of estimates. The observed variance of this set is the bootstrap estimate of variance. The difference between the average of the set of estimates and the original estimate is the bootstrap estimate of bias.

BREAKPOINT In helminth epidemiology, the critical mean wormload in a community, below which the helminth mating frequency is too low to maintain reproduction. A value exceeding the breakpoint of a wormload means that the wormload will increase until equilibrium is reached; a value less than or equal to the breakpoint means that the wormload will decrease progressively.

BYTE A group of adjacent bits, commonly 4, 6, or 8, operating as a unit for storage and manipulation of data in a computer. See also BIT.

C

CALIPER MATCHING see MATCHING.

CANADIAN MORTALITY DATA BASE A large set of computer-stored death statistics; personal identifiers and causes of all deaths in Canada since 1950 have been computer-stored, and the death certificates have been preserved on microfiche. This data base and record linkage have been used in some important historical cohort studies. See also NATIONAL DEATH INDEX.

CANCER REGISTRY See REGISTER.

CARRIER

1. A person or animal that harbors a specific infectious agent in the absence of discernible clinical disease and serves as a potential source of infection. The carrier state may occur in an individual with an infection that is inapparent throughout its course (known as healthy or asymptomatic carrier), or during the incubation period, convalescence, and postconvalescence of an individual with a clinically recognizable disease (known as incubatory carrier or convalescent carrier). The carrier state may be of short or long duration (temporary or transient carrier or chronic carrier).[1]

[1] Adapted from *Control of Communicable Disease in Man,* 14th ed. Washington, DC: American Public Health Association, 1985.

CARRYING CAPACITY An estimate of the numbers of people that a nation, region, or the planet can sustain.

CASE In epidemiology, a person in the population or study group identified as having the particular disease, health disorder, or condition under investigation. A variety of criteria may be used to identify cases, e.g., individual physicians' diagnoses, registries and notifications, abstracts of clinical records, surveys of the general population, population screening, and reporting of defects such as in a dental record. The epidemiologic definition of a case is not necessarily the same as the ordinary clinical definition.

CASE-BASE STUDY A study that starts with the identification and sampling of persons with the disease of interest, and then samples the entire base population (of cases and noncases) from which the original cases arose. This design is similar to a CASE CONTROL STUDY in most respects, but cases may appear in the comparison (base) sample as well as in the case sample.

CASE, COLLATERAL A case occurring in the immediate vicinity of a case which has been the subject of an epidemiological investigation; a term used mainly in malaria control programs, equivalent to the term contact as used in infectious disease epidemiology.

CASE COMPARISON STUDY See CASE CONTROL STUDY.

CASE COMPEER STUDY See CASE CONTROL STUDY.

CASE CONTROL STUDY (Syn: case comparison study, case compeer study, case history study, case referent study, retrospective study) A study that starts with the identification of persons with the disease (or other outcome variable) of interest, and a suitable control (comparison, reference) group of persons without the disease. The relationship of an attribute to the disease is examined by comparing the diseased and nondiseased with regard to how frequently the attribute is present or, if quantitative, the levels of the attribute, in each of the groups.

Such a study can be called "retrospective" because it starts after the onset of disease and looks back to the postulated causal factors. Cases and controls in a case control study may be accumulated "prospectively;" that is, as each new case is diagnosed it is entered in the study. Nevertheless, such a study may still be called "retrospective" because it looks back from the outcome to its causes. The terms "cases" and "controls" are sometimes used to describe subjects in a RANDOMIZED CONTROLLED TRIAL but, the term "case control study" should not be used to describe such a study.

The terms "case control study" and "retrospective study" have been used most often to describe this method. Other terms also used are listed above. The concept of the case-control study is to be found in the works of P.C.A. Louis;[1] the first explicit description of the method is contained in a paper by William Augustus Guy, who reported his analysis of the relationship between prior occupational exposure and the occurrence of pulmonary consumption to the Statistical Society of London in 1843.[2] The evolution of the case-control study thereafter has been described by Lilienfeld and Lilienfeld.[3] The first modern use of the method was a case-control study of breast cancer, reported by Lane-Claypon[4] in 1926; from that time onward, case-control studies became increasingly popular and widely used.

[1]Louis PCA: Researches on Phthisis; Anatomical, Pathological and Therapeutical. (Trans. W.H. Wolshe). London: Sydenham Society, 1844.

[2]Guy WA: Contributions to a knowledge of the influence of employments on health. *J Roy Stat Soc* 6:197–211, 1843.

[3]Lilienfeld AM, Lilienfeld D: A century of case-control studies—progress. *J Chron Dis* 32:5–13, 1979.

[4]Lane-Claypon JE: A further report on cancer of the breast. *Rept Pub Hlth Med Subj* 32. London: HMSO, 1926.

CASE FATALITY RATE The proportion of cases of a specified condition which are fatal within a specified time.

$$\text{Case fatality rate (usually expressed as a percentage)} = \frac{\text{Number of deaths from a disease (in a given period)}}{\text{Number of diagnosed cases of that disease (in the same period)}} \times 100$$

This definition can lead to paradox when more persons die of the disease than develop it during a given period. For instance, chemical poisoning that is slowly but inexorably fatal may cause many persons to develop the disease over a relatively short period of time, but the deaths may not occur until some years later and may be spread over a period of years during which there are no new cases. Thus, in calculating the case fatality rate, it is necessary to acknowledge that the time dimension varies: it may be brief, e.g., covering only the period of stay in a hospital, of finite duration, e.g., one year, or of longer duration still. The term "case fatality rate" is then better replaced by a term such as "survival rate" or by the use of a SURVIVORSHIP TABLE. See also ATTACK RATE.

CASE HISTORY STUDY
1. Synonym for CASE CONTROL STUDY.
2. In clinical medicine, a case report, or a report on a series of cases.

CASE REFERENT STUDY See CASE CONTROL STUDY.

CATASTROPHE THEORY A branch of mathematics dealing with large changes in the total system that may result from small changes in a critical variable in the system. An example is the sudden change in the physical state of water into steam or ice with rise or fall of temperature beyond a critical level. Certain epidemics, gene frequencies, and behavioral phenomena in populations may abide by the same mathematical rule. Herd immunity is an example.

CATCHMENT AREA Region, which may be well- or ill-defined, from which the clients of a particular health facility are drawn.

CAUSALITY The relating of causes to the effects they produce. Most of epidemiology concerns causality and several types of causes can be distinguished. It should be clearly stated, however, that epidemiologic evidence by itself is insufficient to establish causality.

A cause is termed "necessary" when it must always precede an effect. This effect need not be the sole result of the one cause. A cause is termed "sufficient" when it inevitably initiates or produces an effect. Any given cause may be necessary, sufficient, neither, or both. These possibilities are explained below.

Four conditions under which independent variable X may cause Y

	variable X may cause Y	
	X is necessary	X is sufficient
1.	+	+
2.	+	−
3.	−	+
4.	−	−

1. X is necessary and sufficient to cause Y. Both X and Y are always present together, and nothing but X is needed to cause Y; $X \rightarrow Y$.
2. X is necessary but not sufficient to cause Y. X must be present when Y is present, but Y is not always present when X is. Some additional factor(s) must also be present; X and $Z \rightarrow Y$.
3. X is not necessary but is sufficient to cause Y. Y is present when X is, but X may or may not be present when Y is present, because Y has other causes and can occur without X. For example, an enlarged spleen can have many separate causes that are unconnected with each other; $X \rightarrow Y$; $Z \rightarrow Y$.
4. X is neither necessary nor sufficient to cause Y. Again, X may or may not be present when Y is present. Under these conditions, however, if X is present with Y, some additional factor must also be present. Here X is a contributory cause of Y in some causal sequences; X and $Z \rightarrow Y$; W and $Z \rightarrow Y$. These relationships and the logic of causal inference are discussed in *Causal Inference*.[1]

[1] Rothman KJ (Ed): *Causal Inference*. Chestnut Hill, MA: Epidemiology Resources Inc., 1988.

CAUSATION OF DISEASE, FACTORS IN The following factors have been differentiated (but they are not mutually exclusive):

Predisposing factors are those that prepare, sensitize, condition, or otherwise create a situation such as a level of immunity or state of susceptibility so that the host tends to react in a specific fashion to a disease agent, personal interaction, environmental stimulus, or specific incentive. Examples include age, sex, marital status, family size, educational level, previous illness experience, presence of concurrent illness, dependency, working environment, and attitudes toward the use of health services. These factors may be "necessary" but are rarely "sufficient" to cause the phenomenon under study.

Enabling factors are those that facilitate the manifestation of disease, disability, ill-health, or the use of services or conversely those that facilitate recovery from illness, maintenance or enhancement of health status, or more appropriate use of health services. Examples include income, health insurance coverage, nutrition, climate, housing, personal support systems, and availability of medical care. These factors may be "necessary" but are rarely "sufficient" to cause the phenomenon under study.

Precipitating factors are those associated with the definitive onset of a disease, illness, accident, behavioral response, or course of action. Usually one factor is more important or more obviously recognizable than others if several are involved and one may often be regarded as "necessary." Examples include exposure to specific disease, amount or level of an infectious organism, drug, noxious agent, physical trauma, personal interaction, occupational stimulus, or new awareness or knowledge.

Reinforcing factors are those tending to perpetuate or aggravate the presence of a disease, disability, impairment, attitude, pattern of behavior, or course of action. They may tend to be repetitive, recurrent, or persistent and may or may not necessarily be the same or similar to those categorized as predisposing, enabling, or precipitating. Examples include repeated exposure to the same noxious stimulus (in the absence of an appropriate immune response) such as an infectious agent, work, household, or interpersonal environment, presence of financial incentive or disincentive, personal satisfaction, or deprivation.

CAUSES OF DEATH See DEATH CERTIFICATE.

CAUSE-DELETED LIFE TABLE A life table constructed using death rates lowered by eliminating the risk of dying from a specified cause; its most common use is to calculate the gain in life expectancy that would result from the elimination of one cause.

CAUSE-SPECIFIC RATE A rate that specifies events, such as deaths, according to their cause.

CENSORING This term refers to the loss of subjects from a follow-up study; the occurrence of the event of interest among such subjects is uncertain after a specified time when it was known that the event of interest had *not* occurred; it is not known, however, if or when the event of interest occurred subsequently. Such subjects are described as censored. For example, in a follow-up study with myocardial infarction as the outcome of interest, a subject who has not had an infarct but is killed in a traffic crash in year 6 is described as censored as of year 6, since it cannot be known when, if ever, he might have had an infarct at a later year of follow-up. This is censoring by competing risk; other varieties include loss to follow-up and termination of the study. Examination of data for censoring requires the use of special analytic methods, such as life table analysis.

CENSUS An enumeration of a population, originally intended for purposes of taxation and military service. Census enumeration of a population usually records identities of all persons in every place of residence, with age, or birth date, sex, occupation, national origin, language, marital status, income, and relationship to head of household, in addition to information on the dwelling place. Many other items of information may be included, e.g., educational level (or literacy), and health-related data such as permanent disability. A de facto census allocates persons according to their location at the time of enumeration. A de jure census assigns persons according to their usual place of residence at the time of enumeration.

CENSUS TRACT An area for which details of population structure are separately tabulated at a periodic census; normally it is the smallest unit of analysis of (published) census tabulations. Census tracts are chosen because they have well-defined boundaries, sometimes the same as local political jurisdictions, sometimes defined by conspicuous geographical features such as main roads, rivers. In urban areas census tracts may be further subdivided, e.g., into city blocks, but published tables do not contain details to this level.

CENTILE see QUANTILES.

CESSATION EXPERIMENT Controlled study in which an attempt is made to evaluate the termination of an exposure to risk such as a living habit that is considered to be of etiologic importance.

CHART The medical dossier of a patient. See also INFORMATION SYSTEM; MEDICAL RECORD.

CHECK DIGIT A single digit, derived from a multidigit number such as a case identification number, that is used as a screening test for transcription errors.

CHEMOPROPHYLAXIS The administration of a chemical, including antibiotics, to prevent the development of an infection or the progression of an infection to active manifest disease.

CHEMOTHERAPY The use of a chemical to treat a clinically recognizable disease or to limit its further progress.

CHILD DEATH RATE The number of deaths of children aged 1–4 years in a given year per 1000 children in this age group. This is a useful measure of the burden of preventable communicable diseases in the child population.

CHI-SQUARE (χ^2) DISTRIBUTION A variable is said to have a chi-square distribution with K degrees of freedom if it is distributed like the sum of the squares of K independent random variables, each of which has a normal distribution with mean zero and variance one.

CHI-SQUARE (χ^2) TEST Any statistical test based on comparison of a test statistic to a chi-square distribution. The oldest and most common chi-square tests are for detecting whether two or more population distributions differ from one another; these tests usually involve counts of data, and may involve comparison of samples from the distributions under study, or the comparison of a sample to a theoretically expected distribution. The Pearson chi-square test is probably the best known; another is the Mantel–Haenszel test. (Statisticians disagree about the terminal letter; a bare majority of those who contributed to the discussion of this entry prefer "chi-square" rather than "chi-squared." Either usage is acceptable.)

CHRISOMS This word, which appears in BILLS OF MORTALITY, means infants who die before formal baptism; therefore, the number recorded in Bills of Mortality can be used to estimate (albeit inaccurately) neonatal death rates in studies of historical demography and epidemiology.

CHRONIC 1. Referring to a health-related state, lasting a long time. 2. Referring to exposure, prolonged or long-term, often with specific reference to low-intensity. 3. The U.S. National Center for Health Statistics defines a "chronic" condition as one of three months' duration or longer.

CLASS A term used in the theory of frequency distributions. The total number of observations made upon a particular variate may be grouped into classes according to convenient divisions of the variate range in order to make subsequent analyses less laborious, or for other reasons. A group so determined is called a "class." The variate values that determine the upper and lower limits of a class are called "class boundaries," the interval between them is the class interval, and the frequency falling into the class is the class frequency.

CLASSIFICATION (Syn: categorization) Assignment to predesignated classes on the basis of perceived common characteristics. A means of giving order to a group of disconnected facts. Ideally, a classification should be characterized by (1) naturalness—the classes correspond to the nature of the thing being classified, (2) exhaustiveness—every member of the group will fit into one (and only one) class in the system, (3) usefulness—the classification is practical, (4) simplicity—the subclasses are not excessive, and (5) constructability—the set of classes can be constructed by a demonstrably systematic procedure.

CLASSIFICATION OF DISEASES Arrangement of diseases into groups having common characteristics. Useful in efforts to achieve standardization, and therefore comparability, in the methods of presentation of mortality and morbidity data from different sources. May include a systematic numerical notation for each disease entry.

Examples include the INTERNATIONAL CLASSIFICATION OF DISEASES, INJURIES, AND CAUSES OF DEATH (ICD) and the INTERNATIONAL CLASSIFICATION OF HEALTH PROBLEMS IN PRIMARY CARE (ICHPPC).

CLASS, SOCIAL A method of socially stratifying populations, e.g., according to education, income, or occupation. See also SOCIOECONOMIC CLASSIFICATION.

CLINICAL DECISION ANALYSIS Application of DECISION ANALYSIS in a clinical setting with the aim of applying epidemiologic and other data on probability of outcomes when alternative decisions can be made, e.g., surgical intervention or drug treatment for myocardial ischemia.

CLINICAL EPIDEMIOLOGIST A practitioner of clinical epidemiology.

CLINICAL EPIDEMIOLOGY While some epidemiologists deplore any adjectival qualification of the discipline, a subspecialty of clinical epidemiology is sufficiently demarcated to justify definition. There are plenty of suggested definitions. John R. Paul[1] proposed "A marriage between quantitative concepts used by epidemiologists to study disease in populations and decision-making in the individual case which is the daily fare of clinical medicine." Patient care is central to Sackett's definition[2]: "The application, by a physician who provides direct patient care, of epidemiologic and biometric methods to the study of diagnostic and therapeutic processes in order to effect an improvement in health." While limiting the discipline to medical graduates in clinical practice, this definition is conceptually close to the definition of clinical decision analysis; the proper distinction between clinical epidemiology and clinical decision analysis may be that the epidemiologist works with a defined population, even if it is a population of patients rather than a community-based population with numerator and denominator in the conventional epidemiologic sense; clinical decision analysis can be applied to a single patient. Abramson's definition[3] is "The use of epidemiological principles, methods and findings in personal health care or community-oriented primary care, with special reference to applications in diagnostic and prognostic appraisal, decisions concerning care and the evaluation of care. The term sometimes refers to any epidemiological study conducted in a clinical setting." Weiss[4] defines clinical epidemiology as "The study of variation in the outcome of illness and of the reasons for that variation." The existence of the above and other subtly different definitions suggests that this branch of epidemiology remains inchoate.

[1] *J Clin Invest* 17:539–541, 1938.
[2] *Am J Epidemiol* 89:125–128, 1969.
[3] Personal communication, 1986.
[4] *Clinical Epidemiology.* New York: Oxford University Press, 1986.

CLINICAL TRIAL (Syn: therapeutic trial) A research activity that involves the administration of a test regimen to humans to evaluate its efficacy and safety. The term is subject to wide variation in usage, from the first use in humans without any control treatment to a rigorously designed and executed experiment involving test and control treatments and randomization.

See also COMMUNITY TRIAL.

CLINIMETRICS Feinstein,[1] who coined this term, defines it as the domain concerned with indexes, rating scales, and other expressions that are used to describe or measure symptoms, physical signs, and other distinctly clinical phenomena in clinical medicine. Such measurements, of course, are an essential part of many epidemiologic studies.

[1] Feinstein AR: *Clinimetrics.* New Haven and London: Yale University Press, 1987.

CLOSED COHORT A population in which membership begins at a defined time or with a defined event and ends only through occurrence of the study outcome or the end of eligibility for membership. An example is a population of women in labor being studied to determine the vital status of their offspring (i.e., whether live or stillborn).

CLUSTER ANALYSIS A set of statistical methods used to group variables or observations into strongly interrelated subgroups.

CLUSTERING (Syn: disease cluster, time cluster, time–place cluster) A closely grouped series of events or cases of a disease or other health-related phenomena with well-defined distribution patterns, in relation to time or place or both. The term is normally used to describe aggregation of relatively uncommon events or diseases, e.g., leukemia, multiple sclerosis.

CLUSTER SAMPLING A sampling method in which each unit selected is a group of persons (all persons in a city block, a family, etc.) rather than an individual.

CODING Translation of information, e.g., questionnaire responses, into numbered categories for entry in a data processing system.

COEFFICIENT OF VARIATION The ratio of the standard deviation to the mean. This is meaningful only if the variable is measured on a ratio scale. See MEASUREMENT SCALE.

COHORT [from Latin *cohors,* warriors, the tenth part of a legion]
  1. The component of the population born during a particular period and identified by period of birth so that its characteristics (e.g., causes of death and numbers still living) can be ascertained as it enters successive time and age periods.
  2. The term "cohort" has broadened to describe any designated group of persons who are followed or traced over a period of time, as in COHORT STUDY (prospective study).

COHORT ANALYSIS The tabulation and analysis of morbidity or mortality rates in relationship to the ages of a specific group of people (cohort), identified at a particular period of time and followed as they pass through different ages during part or all of their life span. In certain circumstances, e.g., studies of migrant populations, cohort analysis may be performed according to duration of residence of migrants in a country rather than year of birth, in order to relate health or mortality experience to duration of exposure.

COHORT COMPONENT METHOD A method of population projection that takes the population distributed by age and sex at a base date and carries it forward in time on the basis of separate allowances for fertility, mortality, and migration.

COHORT EFFECT See GENERATION EFFECT.

COHORT INCIDENCE See INCIDENCE.

COHORT SLOPES Arrangement of data so that when plotted graphically, lines connect points representing the age-specific rates for population segments from the same

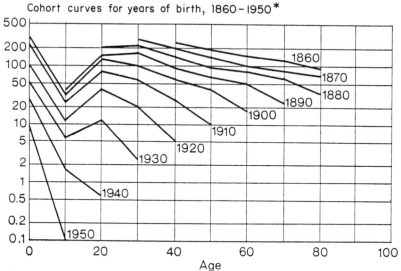

Cohort curves for years of birth, 1860–1950*

* The line associated with each year indicates death rates
by age-group for persons born in that year

Cohort slopes (tuberculosis mortality rates of successive birth generations). Death rates for
tuberculosis, by age, United States, 1900–1960 (per 100,000 population).
From Susser, Watson, Hopper, 1985.

generation of birth (see diagram). These slopes represent changes in rates with age
during the life experience of each cohort.

COHORT STUDY (Syn: concurrent, follow-up, incidence, longitudinal, prospective study)
The method of epidemiologic study in which subsets of a defined population can
be identified who are, have been, or in the future may be exposed or not exposed,
or exposed in different degrees, to a factor or factors hypothesized to influence the
probability of occurrence of a given disease or other outcome. The alternative terms
for a cohort study, i.e., follow-up, longitudinal, and prospective study, describe an
essential feature of the method, which is observation of the population for a sufficient number of person-years to generate reliable incidence or mortality rates in
the population subsets. This generally implies study of a large population, study
for a prolonged period (years), or both.

COINTERVENTION In a RANDOMIZED CONTROLLED TRIAL, the application of additional diagnostic or therapeutic procedures to members of either or both the experimental
and the control groups.

COLD CHAIN A system of protection against high environmental temperatures for heat-
labile vaccines, sera, and other active biological preparations. Unless the cold chain
is preserved, such preparations are inactivated and immunization procedures, etc.
will be ineffective. Preservation of the cold chain is an integral part of the WHO
expanded program on immunization in tropical countries.

COLLINEARITY Very high correlation between variables.

COLONIZATION See INFECTION.

COMMENSAL Literally, eating together (sharing the same table); an organism that lives
harmlessly in the gut. See also XENOBIOTIC.

COMMON SOURCE EPIDEMIC (Syn: common vehicle epidemic) See EPIDEMIC, COMMON
SOURCE.

COMMON VEHICLE SPREAD Spread of disease agent from a source that is common to those who acquire the disease, e.g., water, milk, shellfish, foods, air, or syringe contaminated by infectious or noxious agents. See also TRANSMISSION OF INFECTION.

COMMUNICABLE DISEASE (Syn: infectious disease) An illness due to a specific infectious agent or its toxic products that arises through transmission of that agent or its products from an infected person, animal, or reservoir to a susceptible host, either directly or indirectly through an intermediate plant or animal host, vector, or the inanimate environment. See also TRANSMISSION OF INFECTION.

COMMUNICABLE PERIOD The time during which an infectious agent may be transferred directly or indirectly from an infected person to another person, from an infected animal to man, or from an infected person to an animal, including arthropods. See also TRANSMISSION OF INFECTION.

COMMUNITY A group of individuals organized into a unit, or manifesting some unifying trait or common interest; loosely, the locality or catchment area population for which a service is provided, or more broadly, the state, nation, or body politic.

COMMUNITY DIAGNOSIS The process of appraising the health status of a community, including assembly of vital statistics and other health-related statistics and of information pertaining to determinants of health, such as prevalence of tobacco smoking, and examination of the relationships of these determinants to health in the specified community. The term may also denote the findings of this diagnostic process. Community diagnosis may attempt to be comprehensive, or may be restricted to specific health conditions, determinants, or subgroups. J.N. Morris[1] identified community diagnosis as one of the uses of epidemiology.

[1]*Br Med J* 2:395–401, 1955.

COMMUNITY HEALTH See PUBLIC HEALTH.

COMMUNITY MEDICINE Since the late 1960s, this term has gained wide currency as the preferred name for important activities concerning health care in the community. There are several different definitions, including the following.

1. The field concerned with the study of health and disease in the population of a defined community or group. Its goal is to identify the health problems and needs of defined populations, to identify means by which these needs should be met, and to evaluate the extent to which health services effectively meet these needs.

2. The practice of medicine concerned with groups or populations rather than with individual patients. This includes the elements listed in definition 1, together with the organization and provision of health care at a community or group level.

3. The term is also used to describe the practice of medicine in the community, e.g., by a family physician. Some writers equate the terms "family medicine" and "community medicine"; others confine its use to public health practice.

4. Community-oriented primary health care is an integration of community medicine with the primary health care of individuals in the community. In this form of practice the community practitioner or community health team has responsibility for health care both at a community and at an individual level.

See also PUBLIC HEALTH; SOCIAL MEDICINE.

COMMUNITY TRIAL Experiment in which the unit of allocation to receive a preventive or therapeutic regimen is an entire community or political subdivision. Examples include the trials of fluoridation of drinking water, and of heart disease prevention in North Karelia (Finland) and California. See also CLINICAL TRIAL.

COMORBIDITY Disease(s) that coexist(s) in a study participant in addition to the index condition that is the subject of study.

COMPARISON GROUP Any group to which the index group is compared. Usually synonymous with control group.

COMPETING CAUSE When a previously common cause of death becomes rare, other causes become more prominent. These other causes are referred to as competing causes. For instance, among young adults, pneumonia and other infections were a common cause of death until about midway through the 20th century; their control has brought to prominence some competing causes of death, notably malignant disease and suicide.

COMPETING RISK An event that removes a subject from being at risk for the outcome under investigation. For example, in a study of smoking and cancer of the lung, a subject who dies of coronary heart disease is no longer at risk of lung cancer, and in this situation, coronary heart disease is a competing risk.

COMPLETED FERTILITY RATE The number of children born alive per woman in a cohort of women by the end of their child-bearing years.

COMPLETING THE CLINICAL PICTURE The use of epidemiology to define all modes of presentation of a disease, and/or all possible outcomes. One of the "uses of epidemiology" identified by J.N. Morris.[1]

[1]*Br Med J* 2:395–401, 1955.

COMPLETION RATE The proportion or percentage of persons in a SURVEY for whom complete data are available for analysis. See also RESPONSE RATE.

COMPOSITE INDEX An index, such as the Apgar score, Tumor/Nodes/Metastates (TNM) stage of cancer, that contains contributions from categories of several different variables.

COMPUTER A programmable electronic device that can be used to store and manipulate data in order to carry out designated functions. The two fundamental components of a computer are hardware, i.e., the actual electronic device, and software, the instructions or program used to carry out the function. Computer science has created a large language of its own, describing types of computers (main-frame, micro, digital, analogue, etc.) and all aspects of the process. Most of the terms used in this field are defined by AJ Meadows, M Gordon, and A Singleton.[1]

[1]*Dictionary of New Information Technology.* London: Century, 1982.

CONCORDANCE Pairs or groups of individuals of identical phenotype. In twin studies, a condition in which both twins exhibit or fail to exhibit a trait under investigation.

CONCORDANT A term used in TWIN STUDIES to describe a twin pair in which both twins exhibit a certain trait.

CONCURRENT STUDY See COHORT STUDY.

CONDITIONAL PROBABILITY The probability of an event, given that another event has occurred. If D and E are two events and $P(.\ .\ .)$ is "the probability of $(.\ .\ .)$," the conditional probability of D, given that E occurs, is denoted $P(D|E)$, where the vertical slash is read "given" and is equal to $P(D$ and $E)/P(E)$. The event E is the "conditioning event." Conditional probabilities obey all the axioms of probability theory. See also BAYES' THEOREM; PROBABILITY THEORY.

CONFIDENCE INTERVAL A range of values for a variable of interest, e.g., a rate, constructed so that this range has a specified probability of including the true value of the variable. The specified probability is called the confidence level, and the end points of the confidence interval are called the confidence limits.

CONFOUNDING [from the Latin *confundere*, to mix together]
   1. A situation in which the effects of two processes are not separated. The dis-

tortion of the apparent effect of an exposure on risk brought about by the association with other factors that can influence the outcome.

2. A relationship between the effects of two or more causal factors as observed in a set of data, such that it is not logically possible to separate the contribution that any single causal factor has made to an effect.

3. A situation in which a measure of the effect of an exposure on risk is distorted because of the association of exposure with other factor(s) that influence the outcome under study.

CONFOUNDING VARIABLE (Syn: confounder) A variable that can cause or prevent the outcome of interest, is not an intermediate variable, and is not associated with the factor under investigation. Such a variable must be controlled in order to obtain an undistorted estimate of the effect of the study factor on risk.

CONSANGUINE Related by a common ancestor within the previous few generations.

CONSISTENCY

1. Close conformity between the findings in different samples, strata, or populations, or at different times or in different circumstances, or in studies conducted by different methods or different investigators. Consistency may be examined in order to study effect modification. Consistency of results on replication of studies is an important criterion in judgments of causality.

2. In statistics, an estimator is said to be consistent if the probability of it yielding estimates close to the true value approaches one as the sample size grows larger.

CONTACT (OF AN INFECTION) A person or animal that has been in such association with an infected person or animal or a contaminated environment as to have had opportunity to acquire the infection.

CONTACT, DIRECT A mode of transmission of infection between an infected host and susceptible host. Direct contact occurs when skin or mucous surfaces touch, as in shaking hands, kissing, and sexual intercourse. See also CONTAGION; TRANSMISSION OF INFECTION.

CONTACT, INDIRECT A mode of transmission of infection involving FOMITES or VECTORS. Vectors may be mechanical (e.g., filth flies) or biological (the disease agent undergoes part of its life cycle in the vector species). See also TRANSMISSION OF INFECTION.

CONTACT, PRIMARY Person(s) in direct contact or associated with a communicable disease case.

CONTACT, SECONDARY Person(s) in contact or associated with a primary contact.

CONTAGION The transmission of infection by direct contact, droplet spread, or contaminated FOMITES. These are the modes of transmission specified by FRACASTORIUS in *De Contagione* (1546); contemporary usage is sometimes looser, but use of this term is best restricted to description of infection transmitted by direct contact.

CONTAGIOUS Transmitted by contact; in common usage, "highly infectious."

CONTAINMENT The concept of regional eradication of communicable disease, first proposed by Soper in 1949 for the elimination of smallpox.[1] Containment of a worldwide communicable disease demands a globally coordinated effort so that countries that have effected an interruption of transmission do not become reinfected following importation from neighboring endemic areas.

[1] Pan American Health Organization, OSP, CE7, W-15, Washington DC, 1949.

CONTAMINATION

1. The presence of an infectious agent on a body surface; also on or in clothes, bedding, toys, surgical instruments or dressings, or other inanimate articles or substances including water, milk, and food. Pollution is distinct from contamination and implies the presence of offensive, but not necessarily infectious,

matter in the environment. Contamination of a body surface does not imply a carrier state. See also TRANSMISSION OF INFECTION.

2. The situation that exists when a population being studied for one condition or factor also possesses other conditions or factors that modify results of the study. In a RANDOMIZED CONTROLLED TRIAL, the inadvertent application of the experimental procedure to members of the control group, or inadvertent failure to apply the procedure to members of the experimental group.

CONTINGENCY TABLE A tabular cross-classification of data such that subcategories of one characteristic are indicated horizontally (in rows) and subcategories of another characteristic are indicated vertically (in columns). Tests of association between the characteristics in the columns and rows can be readily applied. The simplest contingency table is the fourfold, or 2×2 table. Contingency tables may be extended to include several dimensions of classification.

CONTINGENT VARIABLE See INTERMEDIATE VARIABLE.

CONTINUING SOURCE EPIDEMIC (OUTBREAK) An epidemic in which new cases of disease occur over a long period, indicating persistence of the disease source.

CONTINUOUS DATA, CONTINUOUS VARIABLE Data (variable) with a potentially infinite number of possible values along a continuum. Data representing a continuous variable include height, weight, and enzyme output.

CONTROL

1. (v.) To regulate, restrain, correct, restore to normal.
2. (n. or adj.) Applied to many communicable and some noncommunicable conditions, "control" means ongoing operations or programs aimed at reducing the incidence and/or prevalence, or eliminating such conditions.
3. (n.) As used in the expressions case-control study and randomized control(led) trial, "control" means person(s) in a comparison group that differs, respectively, in disease experience or allocation to a regimen, from the subjects of the study.
4. (v.) In statistics, "control" means to adjust for or take into account extraneous influences or observations.
5. (adj.) In the expression "control variable" we refer to an independent variable other than the hypothetical causal variable that has a potential effect on the dependent variable and is subject to control by analysis.

The use of the noun "control" to describe the comparison groups in a case control study and in a randomized control(led) trial can confuse the uninitiated, e.g., ethical review committees; the essential ethical distinction is that there may be no intervention in the lives or health status of the controls in a case-control study, whereas controls in a randomized controlled trial may be asked to undergo a procedure or regimen that may affect their health; their informed consent is therefore essential. Consent may not be required (save to gain access to medical records) to study controls in a case-control study. As M.W. Susser[1] has pointed out, the use of the word "control" as verb, adjective, and noun may confuse even careful readers. The verb is best used in the sense of controlling sources of extraneous variation in the dependent variable, whether by design or analysis. The verb is also used in the sense of controlling disease or its causes. The adjective is best used to describe control variables in contradistinction to uncontrolled and confounding variables. The adjective also can be used to describe a control group assembled for comparison with a group of cases or with an experimental group. The noun is best used to designate the members of a control group.

[1] *Causal Thinking in the Health Sciences.* New York: Oxford, 1973.

CONTROLS, HISTORICAL Persons or patients used for comparison who had the condition or treatment under study at a different time, generally at an earlier period than the study group or cases. Historical controls are often unsatisfactory because other factors affecting the condition under study may have changed to an unknown extent in the time elapsed.

CONTROLS, HOSPITAL Persons used for comparison who are drawn from the population of patients in a hospital. Hospital controls are often a source of SELECTION BIAS.

CONTROLS, MATCHED Controls who are selected so that they are similar to the study group, or cases, in specific characteristics. Some commonly used matching variables are age, sex, race, and socioeconomic status. See also MATCHING.

CONTROLS, NEIGHBORHOOD Persons used for comparison who live in the same locality as cases and therefore may resemble cases in environmental and socioeconomic criteria.

CONTROLS, SIBLING Persons used for comparison who are the siblings of cases and therefore share genetic makeup.

COORDINATES In a two-dimensional graph, the values of ordinate and abscissa that define the locus or position of a point.

CORDON SANITAIRE The barrier erected around a focus of infection. Used mainly in the isolation procedures applied to exclude cases and contacts of life-threatening communicable diseases from society. Mainly of historical interest.

CORRELATION The degree to which variables change together.

CORRELATION COEFFICIENT A measure of association that indicates the degree to which two variables have a linear relationship. This coefficient, represented by the letter r, can vary between $+1$ and -1; when $r = +1$, there is a perfect positive linear relationship in which one variable varies directly with the other; when $r = -1$, there is a perfect negative linear relationship between the variables. The measure can be generalized to quantify the degree of linear relationship between one variable and several others, in which case it is known as the multiple correlation coefficient. Kendall's Tau, Spearman's Rank Correlation, and Pearson's Product Moment Correlation tests are special varieties with occasional applications in epidemiology. M.G. Kendall and W.R. Buckland's *Dictionary of Statistical Terms*[1] gives details.

[1] London: Longman, 1983.

CORRELATION, NONSENSE A meaningless correlation between two variables. Nonsense correlations sometimes occur when social, economic, or technological changes have the same trend over time as incidence or mortality rates. An example is correlation between the birth rate and the density of storks in parts of Holland and Germany. See also CONFOUNDING; ECOLOGICAL FALLACY.

COST–BENEFIT ANALYSIS An economic analysis in which the costs of medical care and the loss of net earnings due to death or disability are considered. The general rule for the allocation of funds in a cost–benefit analysis is that the ratio of marginal benefit (the benefit of preventing an additional case) to marginal cost (the cost of preventing an additional case) should be equal to or greater than 1.

COST–EFFECTIVENESS ANALYSIS This form of analysis seeks to determine the costs and effectiveness of an activity, or to compare similar alternative activities to determine the relative degree to which they will obtain the desired objectives or outcomes. The preferred action or alternative is one that requires the least cost to produce a given level of effectiveness, or provides the greatest effectiveness for a given level of cost. In the health care field, outcomes are measured in terms of health status.

COST–UTILITY ANALYSIS An economic analysis in which outcomes are measured in terms of their social value.

COVARIATE A variable that is possibly predictive of the outcome under study. A covariate may be of direct interest to the study or may be a confounding variable or effect modifier.

COVERAGE A measure of the extent to which the services rendered cover the potential need for these services in a community. It is expressed as a proportion in which the numerator is the number of services rendered, and the denominator is the number of instances in which the service should have been rendered. Example:

$$\text{Annual obstetric coverage in a community} = \frac{\text{Number of deliveries attended by a qualified midwife or obstetrician}}{\text{Expected number of deliveries during the year in a given community}}$$

COX MODEL See PROPORTIONAL HAZARDS MODEL.

CRITERION A principle or standard by which something is judged. See also STANDARD.

CRONBACH'S ALPHA (Syn: internal consistency reliability) An estimate of the correlation between the total score across a series of items from a rating scale and the total score that would have been obtained had a comparable series of items been employed.

CROSS-CULTURAL STUDY A study in which populations from different cultural backgrounds are compared.

CROSSOVER DESIGN A method of comparing two or more treatments or interventions in which the subjects or patients, upon completion of the course of one treatment, are switched to another. In the case of two treatments, A and B, half the subjects are randomly allocated to receive these in the order A, B and half to receive them in the order B, A. A criticism of this design is that effects of the first treatment may carry over into the period when the second is given.

CROSS-PRODUCT RATIO See ODDS RATIO.

CROSS-SECTIONAL STUDY (Syn: disease frequency survey, prevalence study) A study that examines the relationship between diseases (or other health-related characteristics) and other variables of interest as they exist in a defined population at one particular time. The presence or absence of disease and the presence or absence of the other variables (or, if they are quantitative, their level) are determined in each member of the study population or in a representative sample at one particular time. The relationship between a variable and the disease can be examined (1) in terms of the prevalence of disease in different population subgroups defined according to the presence or absence (or level) of the variables and (2) in terms of the presence or absence (or level) of the variables in the diseased versus the nondiseased. Note that disease prevalence rather than incidence is normally recorded in a cross-sectional study. The temporal sequence of cause and effect cannot necessarily be determined in a cross-sectional study. See also MORBIDITY SURVEY.

CRUDE DEATH RATE See DEATH RATE.

CUMULATIVE DEATH RATE The proportion of a group that dies over a specified time interval. It may refer to all deaths or to deaths from specific cause(s). If follow-up is not complete on all persons the proper estimation of this rate requires the use of methods that take account of CENSORING. Distinct from FORCE OF MORTALITY.

CUMULATIVE INCIDENCE, CUMULATIVE INCIDENCE RATE The number or proportion of a group of people who experience the onset of a health-related event during a specified time interval; this interval is generally the same for all members of the group, but, as in lifetime incidence, it may vary from person to person without reference to age.

CUMULATIVE INCIDENCE RATIO The ratio of the cumulative incidence rate in the exposed to the cumulative incidence rate in the unexposed.

CUSUM Acronym for cumulative sum (of a series of measurements). This is a useful way to demonstrate a change in trend or direction of a series of measurements.[1] Calculation begins with a reference figure, e.g. the expected average measurement. As each new measurement is observed, the reference figure is subtracted, and a cumulative total is produced by adding each successive difference. This cumulative total is the cusum.

[1] Alderson M: An Introduction to Epidemiology, 2nd ed. London: Macmillan, 1983.

CYCLICITY, SEASONAL The annual cycling of incidence on a seasonal basis. Certain acute infectious diseases, if of greater than rare occurrence, peak in one season of the year and reach the low point six months later (or in the opposite season). The onset of some symptoms of some chronic diseases also may show this amplitudinal cyclicity. Demographic phenomena such as marriage and births, and mortality from all causes and certain specific causes, may also exhibit seasonal cyclicity.

CYCLICITY, SECULAR Long-term (greater than one year) cycling of disease incidence. For example, measles in a large, unimmunized population has a high incidence every second year; hepatitis A has a higher incidence every seventh year. Such cycling is the result of continuous exhaustion and replacement of susceptibles in a relatively stable population. Secular cyclicity may have large interval swings as in the recurrence of pandemics of influenza.

CYST COUNT See WORM COUNT.

D

DATA DREDGING A jargon term, meaning analyses done on a post hoc basis without benefit of prestated hypotheses, as a means of identifying noteworthy differences. Such analyses are sometimes done when data have been collected on a large number of variables and hypotheses are suggested by the data; the scientific validity of data dredging is at best dubious, usually unacceptable.

DATA PROCESSING Conversion (as by computer) of crude information into usable or storable form. Data generated by epidemiologic studies are usually transferred to punch cards or optical mark-sense forms and thence to a computer for storage and retrieval. The term is often loosely used to mean also the statistical analysis of data by a computer program. See also PUNCH CARD.

DEATH CERTIFICATE A vital record signed by a licensed physician or, in some nations, by another designated health worker, that includes cause of death, decedent's name, sex, birthdate, and place of residence and of death. Occupation, birthplace, and other information may be included. Immediate cause of death is recorded on the first line, followed by conditions giving rise to the immediate cause; the underlying cause is entered last. The underlying cause is coded and tabulated in official publications of cause-specific mortality. Other significant conditions may also be re-

CAUSE OF DEATH		Approximate interval between onset and death
I		
Disease or condition directly leading to death*	(a)	....
	due to (or as a consequence of)	
Antecedent causes Morbid conditions, if any, giving rise to the above cause, stating the underlying condition last	(b)	....
	due to (or as a consequence of)	
	(c)	
II		
Other significant conditions contributing to the death, but not related to the disease or condition causing it	....	....
	....	....
* This does not mean the mode of dying, e.g., heart failure, asthenia, etc. It means the disease, injury, or complication which caused death.		

International Standard Death Certificate.

corded separately, as is the mode of death, whether accidental or violent, etc. The most important entries on a death certificate are underlying causes of death and cause of death. These are defined in the *Ninth* (1975) *Revision of the International Classification of Diseases,* as follows:

Causes of death: The causes of death to be entered on the medical certificate of cause of death are all those diseases, morbid conditions, or injuries that either resulted in or contributed to death and the circumstances of the accident or violence which produced any such injuries.

Underlying cause of death: The underlying cause of death is (1) the disease or injury that initiated the train of events leading to death, or (2) the circumstances of the accident or violence that produced the fatal injury.

Personal identifying information such as birthplace, parents' names (last name at birth), and birthdates are included on death certificates in some jurisdictions; this extra information makes possible a range of RECORD LINKAGE studies.

DEATH RATE An estimate of the proportion of a population that dies during a specified period. The numerator is the number of persons dying during the period; the denominator is the size of the population, usually estimated as the mid-year population. The death rate in a population is generally calculated by the formula

$$\frac{\text{Number of deaths during a specified period}}{\text{Number of persons at risk of dying during the period}} \times 10^n$$

This rate is an estimate of the person-time death rate, i.e., the death rate per 10^n person-years. If the rate is low, it is also a good estimate of the cumulative death rate. This rate is also called the crude death rate.

DEATH REGISTRATION AREA A geographic area for which mortality data are published.

DECISION ANALYSIS A derivative of operations research and game theory that involves identifying all available choices and potential outcomes of each, in a series of decisions that have to be made about aspects of patient care—diagnostic procedures, therapeutic regimens, prognostic expectations. Epidemiologic data play a large part in determining the probabilities of outcomes following each choice that has to be made. The range of choices can be plotted on a decision tree, and at each branch, or decision node, the probabilities of each outcome that can be predicted are displayed. The decision tree thus portrays the choices available to those responsible for patient care and the probabilities of each outcome that will follow the choice of a particular action or strategy in patient care. The relative worth of each outcome is preferably also described as a utility or quality of life, e.g., a probability of life expectancy or of freedom from disability.[1]

[1] Pauker SG, Kassirer JP: Decision analysis. *N Engl J Med* 316:250–258, 1987.

DECISION TREE The alternative choices expressed in quantitative terms, available at each stage in the process of thinking through a problem, may be likened to branches, and the hierarchical sequence of options, to a tree. Hence, decision tree. It is a graphic device used in DECISION ANALYSIS, in which a series of decision options are represented as branches and subsequent possible outcomes are represented as further branches. The decisions and the eventualities are presented in the order they are likely to occur. The junction where a decision must be taken is called a decision node.

DEDUCTION Reasoned argument proceeding from the general to the particular.

DEGREES OF FREEDOM *(df)* The number of independent comparisons that can be made between the members of a sample. This important concept in statistical testing cannot be defined briefly. It refers to the number of independent contributions to a sampling distribution (such as χ^2, t, and F distribution). In a CONTINGENCY TABLE it is one less than the number of row categories multiplied by one less than the number of column categories.

DEMAND (FOR HEALTH SERVICES) Willingness and/or ability to seek, use, and, in some settings, to pay for services. Sometimes further subdivided into *expressed demand* (equated with use) and *potential demand,* or NEED.

DEMOGRAPHIC TRANSITION The transition from high to low fertility and mortality rates, usually related to technological change and industrialization.

DEMOGRAPHY The study of populations, especially with reference to size and density, fertility, mortality, growth, age distribution, migration, and VITAL STATISTICS, and the interaction of all these with social and economic conditions.

DEMONSTRATION MODEL An experimental health care facility, program, or system with built-in provision for measuring aspects such as costs per unit of service, rates of use by patients or clients, and outcomes of encounters between providers and users. The aim usually is to determine the feasibility, efficacy, effectiveness, and/or efficiency of the model service.

DENOMINATOR The lower portion of a fraction used to calculate a rate or ratio. The population (or population experience, as in person-years, passenger-miles, etc.) at risk in the calculation of a rate or ratio. See also NUMERATOR.

DENSITY OF POPULATION Demographic term meaning numbers of persons in relation to available space.

DENSITY SAMPLING A method of selecting controls in a CASE CONTROL STUDY in which cases are sampled only from incident cases over a specific time period, and controls are sampled and interviewed throughout that period (rather than simply at one point in time, such as the end of the period). This method can reduce bias due to changing exposure patterns in the source population.

DEPENDENCY RATIO Proportion of children and old people in a population in comparison to all others, i.e., the proportion of economically inactive to economically active; "children" are usually defined as ages under 15 and "old people" as ages 65 and over.

DEPENDENT VARIABLE
1. A variable the value of which is dependent on the effect of other variable(s) [independent variable(s)] in the relationship under study. A manifestation or outcome whose variation we seek to explain or account for by the influence of independent variables.
2. In statistics, the dependent variable is the one predicted by a regression equation.

See also INDEPENDENT VARIABLE.

DESCRIPTIVE STUDY A study concerned with and designed only to describe the existing distribution of variables, without regard to causal or other hypotheses. Contrast analytic study. An example is a community health survey, used to determine the health status of the people in a community. Descriptive studies, e.g., analyses of cancer registry data, can be used to measure risks.

DESIGN See RESEARCH DESIGN.

DESIGN VARIABLE
1. A study variable whose distribution in the subjects is determined by the investigator.

2. In statistics, a variable taking on the value 1 to indicate membership in a particular category and 0 or −1 to indicate nonmembership in the category. Used primarily in ANALYSIS OF VARIANCE.

DETERMINANT Any factor, whether event, characteristic, or other definable entity, that brings about change in a health condition, or other defined characteristic. See also CAUSALITY, FACTORS IN.

DIAGNOSIS The process of determining health status and the factors responsible for producing it; may be applied to an individual, family, group, or community. The term is applied both to the process of determination and to its findings. See also DISEASE LABEL.

DIAGNOSTIC INDEX A system for recording diagnoses, diseases, or problems of patients or clients in a medical practice or service, usually including identifying information (name, birthdate, sex) and dates of encounters. See also E-BOOK.

DIFFERENTIAL The difference(s) shown in tabulation of health and vital statistics according to age, sex, or some other factor; age differentials are the differences revealed in the tabulations of rates in age-groups, sex differentials are the differences in rates between males and females, income differentials are differences between designated income categories, etc.

DIGIT PREFERENCE A preference for certain numbers that leads to rounding off measurements. Rounding off may be to the nearest whole number, even number, multiple of 5 or 10, or (when time units like a week are involved) 7, 14, etc. This can be a form of OBSERVER VARIATION, or an attribute of respondent(s) in a survey.

DIMENSIONALITY The number of dimensions, i.e., scalar quantities, needed for accurate description of an element of a vector space.

DIRECT ADJUSTMENT, DIRECT STANDARDIZATION See STANDARDIZATION.

DISABILITY Temporary or long-term reduction of a person's capacity to function in society. See also INTERNATIONAL CLASSIFICATION OF IMPAIRMENTS, DISABILITIES, AND HANDICAPS for the official WHO definition.

DISCORDANT A term used in TWIN STUDIES to describe a twin pair in which one twin exhibits a certain trait and the other does not. Also used in matched pair case control studies to describe a pair whose members had different exposures to the risk factor under study. Only the discordant pairs are informative about the association between exposure and disease.

DISCRETE DATA Data that can be arranged into naturally occurring or arbitrarily selected groups or sets of values, as opposed to data in which there are no naturally occurring breaks in continuity, i.e., CONTINUOUS DATA. An example is number of decayed, missing, and filled teeth (DMF).

DISCRIMINANT ANALYSIS A statistical analytic technique used with discrete dependent variables, concerned with separating sets of observed values and allocating new values; can sometimes be used instead of regression analysis. Kendall and Buckland[1] refer to this as "discriminatory analysis" and describe it as a rule for allocating individuals or values from two or more discrete populations to the correct population with minimal probability of misclassification.

[1] Kendall MG, Buckland WR: *A Dictionary of Statistical Terms*, 4th ed. London: Longman, 1982.

DISEASE Literally, *dis-ease*, the opposite of *ease*, when something is wrong with a bodily function. The words "disease," "illness," and "sickness" are loosely interchangeable, but are better regarded as not wholly synonymous. M. W. Susser has suggested that they be used as follows:

Disease is a physiological/psychological dysfunction.

Illness is a subjective state of the person who feels aware of not being well;

Sickness is a state of social dysfunction, i.e., a role that the individual assumes when ill.

DISEASE FREQUENCY SURVEY See CROSS-SECTIONAL STUDY; MORBITITY SURVEY.

DISEASE LABEL The identity of the condition from which a patient suffers. It may be the name of a precisely defined disorder identified by a battery of tests, a probability statement based on consideration of what is most likely among several possibilities, or an opinion based on pattern recognition. Use of the word "label" can convey stigma, so this term should be used with care, if at all. See also DIAGNOSIS.

DISEASE ODDS RATIO See ODDS RATIO.

DISEASE, PRECLINICAL Disease with no signs or symptoms, because they have not yet developed. See also INAPPARENT INFECTION.

DISEASE REGISTRY See REGISTER, REGISTRY.

DISEASE, SUBCLINICAL A condition in which disease is detectable by special tests but does not reveal itself by signs or symptoms.

DISEASE TAXONOMY See TAXONOMY OF DISEASE.

DISINFECTION Killing of infectious agents outside the body by direct exposure to chemical or physical agents.

Concurrent disinfection is the application of disinfective measures as soon as possible after the discharge of infectious material from the body of an infected person, or after the soiling of articles with such infectious discharges, all personal contact with such discharges or articles being minimized prior to such disinfection.

Terminal disinfection is the application of disinfective measures after the patient has been removed by death or to a hospital, or has ceased to be a source of infection, or after other hospital isolation practices have been discontinued. Terminal disinfection is rarely practiced; terminal cleaning generally suffices, along with airing and sunning of rooms, furniture, and bedding. Disinfection is necessary only for diseases spread by indirect contact; steam sterilization or incineration of bedding and other items is desirable after a disease such as plague or anthrax.[1]

[1] Benenson AS (Ed): *Control of Communicable Diseases in Man,* 14th ed. Washington DC: American Public Health Association 1985.

DISINFESTATION Any physical or chemical process serving to destroy or remove undesired small animal forms, particularly arthropods or rodents, present upon the person, the clothing, or in the environment of an individual, or on domestic animals. Disinfestation includes delousing for infestation with *Pediculus humanus humanus,* the body louse. Synonyms include the terms "disinsection" and "disinsectization" when insects only are involved.

DISTRIBUTION The complete summary of the frequencies of the values or categories of a measurement made on a group of persons. The distribution tells either how many or what proportion of the group was found to have each value (or each range of values) out of all the possible values that the quantitative measure can have.

DISTRIBUTION-FREE METHOD A method which does not depend upon the form of the underlying distribution.

DISTRIBUTION FUNCTION A function that gives the relative frequency with which a random variable falls at or below each of a series of values. Examples include the normal distribution, log-normal distribution, chi-square distribution, t distribution, F-distribution, and binomial distribution, all of which have applications in epidemiology.

DMF The abbreviation DMF stands for decayed, missing, and filled teeth. Lowercase letters, i.e., dmf, are used for deciduous dentition, upper case for permanent teeth. The DMF number is widely used in dental epidemiology.

DOSE–RESPONSE RELATIONSHIP A relationship in which a change in amount, intensity, or duration of exposure is associated with a change—either an increase or a decrease—in risk of a specified outcome.

DOUBLE-BLIND TRIAL A procedure of blind assignment to study and control groups and blind assessment of outcome, designed to ensure that ascertainment of outcome is not biased by knowledge of the group to which an individual was assigned. "Double" refers to both parties, i.e., the observer(s) in contact with the subjects, and the subjects in the study and control groups. See also BLIND EXPERIMENT; RANDOMIZED CONTROLLED TRIAL.

DRIFT See GENETIC DRIFT; SOCIAL DRIFT.

DROPLET NUCLEI A type of particle implicated in the spread of airborne infection. Droplet nuclei are tiny particles (1–10 μm diameter) that represent the dried residue of droplets. They may be formed by (1) evaporation of droplets coughed or sneezed into the air or (2) aerosolization of infective materials. See also TRANSMISSION OF INFECTION.

DROPOUT A person enrolled in a study who becomes inaccessible or ineligible for follow-up, e.g., because of inability or unwillingness to remain enrolled in the study. The occurrence of dropouts can lead to biases in study results.

DUMMY VARIABLE See INDICATOR VARIABLE.

DYNAMIC POPULATION A population that gains and loses members; all natural populations are dynamic, a fact recognized by the term "population dynamics," used by demographers to denote changing composition. See also POPULATION DYNAMICS; STABLE POPULATION.

E

EARLY WARNING SYSTEM In disease surveillance, a specific procedure to detect as early as possible any departure from usual or normally observed frequency of phenomena. For example, the routine monitoring of numbers of deaths from pneumonia and influenza in large American cities is an early warning system for the identification of influenza epidemics. In developing countries, a change in children's average weights is an early warning signal of nutritional deficiency.

E–BOOK Method (developed by Eimerl)[1] of recording encounters in primary medical care: encounters are arranged by problem or diagnostic category, thus making it easy to count the number of persons seen (and the number of times each is seen) according to problem or diagnostic category in a given period of time. Widely used in epidemiologic studies of primary medical care. See also AGE–SEX REGISTER; DIAGNOSTIC INDEX.

[1] Eimerl TS: Organized curiosity. *J Coll Gen Practit* 3:246–252, 1960.

ECOLOGICAL ANALYSIS Analysis based on aggregated or grouped data; errors in inference may result because associations may be artifactually created or masked by the aggregation process.

ECOLOGICAL CORRELATION A correlation in which the units studied are populations rather than individuals. Correlations found in this manner may not hold true for the individual members of these populations. See also ECOLOGICAL FALLACY.

ECOLOGICAL FALLACY (Syn: aggregation bias, ecological bias)
1. The bias that may occur because an association observed between variables on an aggregate level does not necessarily represent the association that exists at an individual level.
2. An error in inference due to failure to distinguish between different levels of organization. A correlation between variables based on group (ecological) characteristics is not necessarily reproduced between variables based on individual characteristics; an association at one level may disappear at another, or even be reversed. Example: At the ecological level, a correlation has been found in several studies between the quality of drinking water and mortality rates from heart disease; it would be an ecological fallacy to infer from this alone that exposure to water of a particular level of hardness necessarily influences the individual's chances of getting or dying of heart disease.

ECOLOGICAL STUDY A study in which the units of analysis are populations or groups of people, rather than individuals. An example is the study of association between median income and cancer mortality rates in administrative jurisdictions such as states and counties.

ECOLOGY The study of the relationships among living organisms and their environment. "Human ecology" means the study of human groups as influenced by environmental factors, often including social and behavioral factors.

ECOSYSTEM The plant and animal life of a region considered in relation to the environmental factors that influence it; more specifically, the fundamental unit in ecology, comprising the living organisms and the nonliving elements that interact in a defined region.

EFFECT The result of a cause. In epidemiology, frequently a synonym for EFFECT MEASURE.

EFFECTIVENESS The extent to which a specific intervention, procedure, regimen, or service, when deployed in the field, does what it is intended to do for a defined population.

EFFECT MEASURE A quantity that measures the effect of a factor on the frequency or risk of a health outcome. Three such measures are attributable fractions, which measure the fraction of cases due to a factor; risk and rate differences, which measure the amount a factor adds to the risk or rate of a disease; and risk and rate ratios, which measure the amount by which a factor multiplies the risk or rate of disease.

EFFECT MODIFIER (Syn: conditional variable, moderator variable) A factor that modifies the effect of a putative causal factor under study. For example, age is an effect modifier for many conditions, and immunization status is an effect modifier for the consequences of exposure to pathogenic organisms. Effect modification is detected by varying the selected effect measure for the factor under study across levels of another factor. See also CAUSALITY, FACTORS IN; INTERACTION.

EFFECTIVE SAMPLE SIZE Sample size after dropouts, deaths, and other specified exclusions from an original sample.

EFFICACY The extent to which a specific intervention, procedure, regimen, or service produces a beneficial result under ideal conditions. Ideally, the determination of efficacy is based on the results of a RANDOMIZED CONTROLLED TRIAL.

EFFICIENCY
1. The effects or end-results achieved in relation to the effort expended in terms of money, resources, and time. The extent to which the resources used to provide a specific intervention, procedure, regimen, or service of known efficacy and effectiveness are minimized. A measure of the economy (or cost in resources) with which a procedure of known efficacy and effectiveness is carried out.
2. In statistics, the relative precision with which a particular study design or estimator will estimate a parameter of interest.

EGG COUNT See WORM COUNT.

ELIMINATION See ERADICATION (OF DISEASE).

EMPIRICAL Based directly on experience, e.g., observation or experiment, rather than on reasoning alone.

ENCOUNTER A face-to-face transaction between a personal health worker and a patient or client.

ENDEMIC DISEASE The constant presence of a disease or infectious agent within a given geographic area or population group; may also refer to the usual prevalence of a given disease within such area or group. See also HOLOENDEMIC DISEASE; HYPERENDEMIC DISEASE.

END RESULTS See OUTCOMES.

ENVIRONMENT All that which is external to the individual human host. Can be divided into physical, biological, social, cultural, etc., any or all of which can influence health status of populations.

EPIDEMIC [from the Greek *epi* (upon), *dēmos* (people)] The occurrence in a community or region of cases of an illness, specific health-related behavior, or other health-related events clearly in excess of normal expectancy. The community or region, and the period in which the cases occur, are specified precisely. The number of cases indicating the presence of an epidemic varies according to the agent, size, and type of population exposed, previous experience or lack of exposure to the disease, and time and place of occurrence; epidemicity is thus relative to usual frequency of the disease in the same area, among the specified population, at the same season of the year. A single case of a communicable disease long absent from a population or first invasion by a disease not previously recognized in that area requires immediate reporting and full field investigation; two cases of such a disease associated in time and place may be sufficient evidence to be considered an epidemic.

The word may be used also to describe outbreaks of disease in animal or plant populations. See also EPIZOOTIC; EPORNITHIC.

EPIDEMIC, COMMON SOURCE (Syn: common vehicle epidemic, holomiantic disease) Outbreak due to exposure of a group of persons to a noxious influence that is common to the individuals in the group. When the exposure is brief and essentially simultaneous, the resultant cases all develop within one incubation period of the disease (a "point" or "point source" epidemic).

The term "holomiantic disease" was used by Stallybrass (1931) to describe outbreaks of this type, but as with several other terms created from Greek or Latin roots, transmission to epidemiologists who lacked a classical education, did not take place.

EPIDEMIC CURVE A graphic plotting of the distribution of cases by time of onset.

EPIDEMIC, MATHEMATICAL MODEL OF See MATHEMATICAL MODEL.

EPIDEMIC, POINT SOURCE See EPIDEMIC, COMMON SOURCE.

EPIDEMIOLOGIST An investigator who studies the occurrence of disease or other health-related conditions or events in defined populations. The control of disease in populations is often also considered to be a task for the epidemiologist, especially in speaking of certain specialized fields such as malaria epidemiology. Epidemiologists may study disease in populations of animals and plants, as well as among human populations. See also CLINICAL EPIDEMIOLOGIST.

EPIDEMIOLOGY The study of the distribution and determinants of health-related states or events in specified populations, and the application of this study to control of health problems.

There have been many definitions of epidemiology. In the past 50 years or so, the definition has broadened from concern with communicable disease epidemics to take in all phenomena related to health in populations.

The *Oxford English Dictionary (OED)* gives as a definition: "That branch of medical science which treats of epidemics" and cites Parkin (1873) as a source. However, there was a "London Epidemiological Society" in the 1850s. The identity of the scholar who first used the word at that time has been lost. *Epidemiologia* appears in the title of a Spanish history of epidemics, *Epidemiologia española*, Madrid, 1802.

Epidemic is much older. The word appears in Johnson's *Dictionary* (1775), and *OED* gives a citation dated 1603. The word was, of course, used by Hippocrates.

EPIDEMIOLOGY, ANALYTIC See ANALYTIC STUDY.

EPIDEMIOLOGY, DESCRIPTIVE Study of the occurrence of disease or other health-related characteristics in human populations, General observations concerning the relationship of disease to basic characteristics such as age, sex, race, occupation, and social class; also concerned with geographic location. The major characteristics in descriptive epidemiology can be classified under the headings: persons, place, and time. See also OBSERVATIONAL STUDY.

EPIDEMIOLOGY, EXPERIMENTAL See EXPERIMENTAL EPIDEMIOLOGY.

EPISODE Period in which a health problem or illness exists, from its onset to its resolution. See also ENCOUNTER.

EPIZOOTIC An outbreak (epidemic) of disease in an animal population (often with the implication that it may also affect human populations).

EPORNITHIC An outbreak (epidemic) of disease in a bird population.

ERADICATION (OF DISEASE) Termination of all transmission of infection by extermination of the infectious agent through surveillance and containment. Eradication, as in the instance of smallpox, was based on the joint activities of control and surveillance. Regional eradication has been successful with malaria and in some countries appears close to succeeding for measles. The term "elimination" is sometimes used to describe eradication of diseases such as measles from a large geographic region or political jurisdiction.

ERROR

1. A false or mistaken result obtained in a study or experiment. Several kinds of error can occur in epidemiology, for example, due to bias.

2. Random error is the portion of variation in a measurement that has no apparent connection to any other measurement or variable, generally regarded as due to chance.

3. Systematic error, which often has a recognizable source, e.g., a faulty measuring instrument, or pattern, e.g., it is consistently wrong in a particular direction. See also BIAS.

ERROR, TYPE I (Syn: alpha error) The error of rejecting a true null hypothesis. See also SIGNIFICANCE LEVEL; STATISTICAL TEST.

ERROR, TYPE II (Syn: beta error) The error of failing to reject a false null hypothesis. See also POWER; STATISTICAL TEST.

ESTIMATE A measurement or a statement about the value of some quantity is said to be an estimate if it is known, believed, or suspected to incorporate some degree of error.

ESTIMATOR In statistics, a function for computing estimates of a parameter from observed data.

ETHICS The branch of philosophy that deals with the distinction between right and wrong, with the moral consequences of human actions. Ethical principles govern the conduct of epidemiology, as they do all human activities; the ethical issues that are specific to epidemiological practice and research include informed consent, confidentiality, and respect for human rights. The issues have been defined, described, and discussed by many writers and by special committees under the auspices of research granting agencies and other official bodies in many countries.[1]

[1]See, for example, the following: Curran WJ: Protecting confidentiality in epidemiologic investigations by the Centers for Disease Control. *N Engl J Med* 314:1027–1028, 1986.

Susser MW, Stein Z, Kline J: Ethics in epidemiology. *Ann Amer Acad Pol Soc Sci* 437:128–141, 1978.

Commonwealth of Australia, National Health and Medical Research Council, Medical Research Ethics Committee: Report on Ethics in Epidemiological Research. Canberra, 1985.

Stolley PD: Faith, evidence and the epidemiologist. *J Public Health Pol* 6:37–42, 1985.

Gordis, L, Gold E, Seltser R: Privacy and protection in epidemiologic and medical research: Challenge and responsiblity. *Am J Epidemiol* 105:163–168, 1977.

National Academy of Sciences, Institute of Medicine: *Ethics of Health Care.* Washington, DC, 1974.

Tancredi LR (ed): Ethical issues in epidemiologic research (Vol. VII, series in Psychosocial Epidemiology). New Brunswick, NJ: Rutgers University Press, 1986.

ETHNIC GROUP A social group characterized by a distinctive social and cultural tradition, maintained within the group from generation to generation, a common history and origin, and a sense of identification with the group. Members of the group have distinctive features in their way of life, shared experiences, and often a common genetic heritage. These features may be reflected in their health and disease experience. See also RACE.

ETIOLOGY Literally, the science of causes, causality; in common usage, cause. See also CAUSALITY; PATHOGENESIS.

ETIOLOGIC FRACTION (EXPOSED) See ATTRIBUTABLE FRACTION (EXPOSED).

ETIOLOGIC FRACTION (POPULATION) See ATTRIBUTABLE FRACTION (POPULATION).

EVALUATION A process that attempts to determine as systematically and objectively as possible the relevance, effectiveness, and impact of activities in the light of their objectives. Several varieties of evaluation can be distinguished, e.g., evaluation of structure, process, and outcome. See also CLINICAL TRIAL; EFFECTIVENESS; EFFICACY; EFFICIENCY; HEALTH SERVICES RESEARCH; PROGRAM EVALUATION AND REVIEW TECHNIQUES; QUALITY OF CARE.

EVAN'S POSTULATES Expanding biomedical knowledge has led to revision of HENLE'S and KOCH'S POSTULATES. Alfred Evans[1] developed those that follow, based on the Henle–Koch model.

1. Prevalence of the disease should be significantly higher in those exposed to the hypothesized cause than in controls not so exposed.
2. Exposure to the hypothesized cause should be more frequent among those with the disease than in controls without the disease—when all other risk factors are held constant.
3. Incidence of the disease should be significantly higher in those exposed to the hypothesized cause than in those not so exposed, as shown by prospective studies.
4. The disease should follow exposure to the hypothesized causative agent with a distribution of incubation periods on a bell-shaped curve.
5. A spectrum of host responses should follow exposure to the hypothesized agent along a logical biological gradient from mild to severe.
6. A measurable host response following exposure to the hypothesized cause should have a high probability of appearing in those lacking this before exposure (e.g., antibody, cancer cells), or should increase in magnitude if present before exposure. This response pattern should occur infrequently in persons not so exposed.
7. Experimental reproduction of the disease should occur more frequently in animals or man appropriately exposed to the hypothesized cause than in those not so exposed; this exposure may be deliberate in volunteers, experimentally induced in the laboratory, or may represent a regulation of natural exposure.
8. Elimination or modification of the hypothesized cause should decrease the incidence of the disease (i.e., attenuation of a virus, removal of tar from cigarettes).
9. Prevention or modification of the host's response on exposure to the hypothesized cause should decrease or eliminate the disease (i.e., immunization, drugs to lower cholesterol, specific lymphocyte transfer factor in cancer).
10. All of the relationships and findings should make biological and epidemiologic sense.

[1] Evans AS: Causation and disease: The Henle–Koch postulates revisited. *Yale J Biol Med* 49:175–195, 1976.

EXACT METHOD A statistical method based on the actual, i.e., "exact" probability distribution of the study data, rather than on an approximation such as the normal or chi-square distribution; for example, Fisher's exact test.

EXACT TEST A statistical test based on the actual null probability distribution of the study data, rather than, say, normal approximation. The most common exact test is the Fisher–Irwin test for fourfold tables.

EXCESS RATE AMONG EXPOSED See RATE DIFFERENCE.

EXCESS RISK A term sometimes used to refer to the POPULATION EXCESS RATE and sometimes to RISK DIFFERENCE.

EXPANDED PROGRAMME ON IMMUNIZATION Part of the effort to achieve "Health for All by the Year 2000," under the auspices of WHO, UNICEF, and other international and bilateral aid agencies. This is a program of immunizing against diphtheria, tetanus, measles, pertussis, poliomyelitis, and tuberculosis, conducted especially in developing countries.

EXPECTATION OF LIFE (Syn: life expectancy or expectation) The average number of years an individual of a given age is expected to live if current mortality rates continue to apply. A statistical abstraction based on existing, age-specific death rates.

Life expectancy at birth $(\mathring{e}_0)$: Average number of years a newborn baby can be expected to live if current mortality trends continue. Corresponds to the total number of years a given birth cohort can be expected to live, divided by the number of children in the cohort. Life expectancy at birth is partly dependent on mortality in the first year of life and is lower in poor than in rich countries because of the higher infant and child mortality rates in the former.

Life expectancy at a given age, age x $(\mathring{e}_x)$: The average number of additional years a person age x would live if current mortality trends continue to apply, based on the age-specific death rates for a given year.

Life expectancy is a hypothetical measure and indicator of current health and mortality conditions. It is not a rate.

EXPERIMENT A study in which the investigator intentionally alters one or more factors under controlled conditions in order to study the effects of so doing.

EXPERIMENTAL EPIDEMIOLOGY In modern usage, this term is often equated with RANDOMIZED CONTROLLED TRIALS. To GREENWOOD and other epidemiologists in the 1920s, it meant the study of epidemics among colonies of experimental animals such as rats and mice. The original meaning of the term is preferable; if the word "experiment" is qualified by the adjective "epidemiologic" it is a synonym for RANDOMIZED CONTROLLED TRIAL. See also ANIMAL MODEL.

EXPERIMENTAL STUDY A study in which conditions are under the direct control of the investigator. In epidemiology, a study in which a population is selected for a planned trial of a regimen whose effects are measured by comparing the outcome of the regimen in the experimental group with the outcome of another regimen in a control group. To avoid BIAS members of the experimental and control groups should be comparable except in the regimen that is offered them. Allocation of individuals to experimental or control groups is ideally by randomization. In a RANDOMIZED CONTROLLED TRIAL, individuals are randomly allocated; in some experiments, e.g., fluoridation of drinking water, whole communities have been (nonrandomly) allocated to experimental and control groups.

EXPLANATORY STUDY A study whose main objective is to explain, rather than merely describe, a situation, by isolating the effects of specific variables and understanding the mechanisms of action. See also PRAGMATIC STUDY.

EXPLANATORY VARIABLE

    1. A variable that causally explains the association or outcome under study.

2. In statistics, a synonym for INDEPENDENT VARIABLE.

EXPOSED In epidemiology, the exposed group (or simply, *the exposed*) is often used to connote a group whose members have been exposed to a supposed cause of a disease or health state of interest, or possess a characteristic that is a determinant of the health outcome of interest.

EXPOSURE

1. Proximity and/or contact with a source of a disease agent in such a manner that effective transmission of the agent or harmful effects of the agent may occur.

2. The amount of a factor to which a group or individual was exposed; sometimes contrasted with dose, the amount that enters or interacts with the organism.

3. Exposures may of course be beneficial rather than harmful, e.g., exposure to immunizing agents.

EXPOSURE-ODDS RATIO See ODDS RATIO.

EXPOSURE RATIO The ratio of rates at which persons in the case and control groups of a CASE CONTROL STUDY are exposed to the RISK FACTOR (or to the protective factor) of interest.

EXPRESSIVITY In genetics, the extent to which a gene is expressed.

EXTRAPOLATE, EXTRAPOLATION To predict the value of a variate outside the range of observations; the resulting prediction. See also INTERPOLATE.

EXTRINSIC INCUBATION PERIOD Time required for development of a disease agent in a vector from the time of uptake of the agent to the time when the vector is infective. See also INCUBATION PERIOD; VECTOR-BORNE INFECTION.

F

F DISTRIBUTION (Syn: Variance ratio distribution) The distribution of the ratio of two independent quantities each of which is distributed like a variance in normally distributed samples. So-named in honor of R.A. Fisher who first described this distribution.

F_1 ("F one") Term used in genetics to describe first-generation progeny of a mating.

FACTOR (Syn: determinant)

1. An event, characteristic, or other definable entity that brings about a change in a health condition or other defined outcome. See also CAUSALITY, CAUSATION OF DISEASE, FACTORS IN.

2. A synonym for (categorical) independent variable, or more precisely, an independent variable used to identify, with numerical codes, membership of qualitatively different groups. A causal role may be implied, as in "overcrowding is a factor in disease transmission" where overcrowding represents the highest level of the factor "crowding."

FACTOR ANALYSIS A set of statistical methods for analyzing the correlations among several variables in order to estimate the number of fundamental dimensions that underlie the observed data and to describe and measure those dimensions. Used frequently in the development of scoring systems for rating scales and questionnaires.

FACTORIAL DESIGN A method of setting up an experiment or study to assure that all levels of each intervention or classificatory factor occur with all levels of the others.

FALSE NEGATIVE Negative test result in a subject who possesses the attribute for which the test is conducted. The labeling of a diseased person as healthy when screening in the detection of disease. See also SCREENING; SENSITIVITY AND SPECIFICITY.

FALSE POSITIVE Positive test result in a subject who does not possess the attribute for which the test is conducted. The labeling of a healthy person as diseased when screening in the detection of disease. See also SCREENING; SENSITIVITY AND SPECIFICITY.

FAMILIAL DISEASE Disease that exhibits a tendency to familial occurrence. Familial occurrence of disease may be due to genetic transmission, intrafamilial transmission of infection or culture, interaction within the family, or the family's shared experience, including its exposure to a common environment.

FAMILY A group of two or more persons united by blood, adoptive or marital ties, or the common law equivalent; the family may include members who do not share the household but are united to other members by blood, adoptive or marital, or equivalent ties. Epidemiologic studies may be concerned with family members or with those who share the same household or dwelling unit.

FAMILY, EXTENDED A group of persons comprising members of several generations united by blood, adoptive and marital, or equivalent ties. See also FAMILY, NUCLEAR.

FAMILY CONTACT DISEASE Disease that occurs among members of the family of a worker who is exposed to a toxic substance and carries this home on his person or his clothing, causing exposure to other family members.

FAMILY, NUCLEAR A group of persons comprising members of a single or at most two generations, usually husband–wife–children, united by blood or adoptive and marital or equivalent ties.

FAMILY OF CLASSIFICATIONS In nosology, a set of related classification systems describing different aspects of health problems. For example, the International Classification of Disease, the International Classification of Health Problems in Primary Care, the International Classification of Impairments, Disabilities and Handicaps, and the specialty subclassifications for oncology, psychiatry, etc. developed by WHO working groups constitute a "family of classifications."

FAMILY STUDY An epidemiologic study of a family or a group of families. The term has been used to describe surveillance of family groups, e.g., for tuberculosis. In genetics, investigation of families showing an unusual characteristic in order to determine whether the characteristic clusters in certain families and if so, why.

FARR, WILLIAM (1807–1883) A medical graduate who became the first compiler of abstracts (statistician) to the Registrar-General in the newly established General Register Office of England in 1839 and remained there for more than 40 years. In his *Annual Reports,* the combination of facts on death rates and vivid language drew attention to many inequalities of health and sickness experience between "healthy" and "unhealthy" districts in England. His many contributions to vital statistics and epidemiology are contained in his monograph *Vital Statistics* (London, 1885). These include a statement of the relationship between incidence and prevalence, the concepts of person-years, retrospective and prospective approaches, observed and expected numbers of events, the first workable NOSOLOGY, and empirical laws about the natural history of epidemics.

FATALITY RATE The death rate observed in a designated series of persons affected by a simultaneous event, e.g., victims of a disaster. A term to be deprecated, because it can be confused with CASE FATALITY RATE.

FEASIBILITY STUDY Preliminary study to determine practicability of a proposed health program or procedure, or of a larger study, and to appraise the factors that may influence its practicability. See also PILOT STUDY.

FECUNDITY The ability to produce live offspring. Fecundity is difficult to measure since it refers to the theoretical ability of a woman to conceive and carry a fetus to term. If a woman produces a live birth, it is known that she and her consort were fecund during some time in the past.

FERTILITY The actual production of live offspring. Stillbirths, fetal deaths, and abortions are not included in the measurement of fertility in a population. See also GRAVIDITY; PARITY.

FERTILITY RATE See GENERAL FERTILITY RATE.

FERTILITY RATIO A measure of the fertility of the population that restricts the denominator to the female population of appropriate age for childbearing. The fertility ratio is defined as

$$\text{Fertility ratio} = \frac{\text{Number of girls under 15 years of age}}{\text{Number of women in 15–49 age group}} \times 1000$$

(Not to be confused with GENERAL FERTILITY RATE.)

FETAL DEATH (Syn: stillbirth) Death prior to the complete expulsion or extraction from its mother of a product of conception, irrespective of the duration of pregnancy. The death is indicated by the fact that after such separation the fetus does not breathe or show any other evidence of life, such as beating of the heart, pulsation of the umbilical cord, or definite movement of voluntary muscles. Defined variously as death after the 20th or 28th week of gestation (the definition of the length of gestation varies between different jurisdictions, making this event difficult to compare internationally). See also LIVE BIRTH.

FETAL DEATH CERTIFICATE (Syn: certificate of stillbirth) A vital record registering a fetal death or stillbirth. Some health jurisdictions require the use of a fetal death certificate for all products of conception, whereas others require its use only in cases in which gestation has reached a particular duration, usually the 20th or the 28th week.

FETAL DEATH RATE (Syn: stillbirth rate) The number of fetal deaths in a year expressed as a proportion of the total number of births (live births plus fetal deaths) in the same year.

$$\text{Fetal death rate} = \frac{\text{Number of fetal deaths in a year}}{\text{Number of fetal deaths plus live births in the same year}} \times 1000$$

Note that the denominator is larger than for the FETAL DEATH RATIO and that the fetal death rate is therefore lower than the fetal death ratio, which is used in some jurisdictions. International comparisons of stillbirth or fetal death statistics will be flawed if the distinction is not appreciated.

FETAL DEATH RATIO A measure of fetal wastage, related to the number of live births. Defined as

$$\text{Fetal death ratio} = \frac{\text{Number of fetal deaths in a year}}{\text{Number of live births in the same year}}$$

(Can be expressed per 1000.)

FIELD SURVEY The planned collection of data in "the field," i.e., usually among noninstitutionalized persons in the general population. A method of establishing a relationship between two or more variables in a population in numerical terms by eliciting and collating information from existing sources (not only records but people who can say how they feel or what happened). See also CROSS-SECTIONAL STUDY.

FINLAY, CARLOS ALBERT (1833–1915) Cuban physician, initial investigator (1888–1891) of the role of *Aedes aegypti* (then known as *Culex fasciatus*) in the transmission of yellow fever. His experiments were unsatisfactory, but his theory was fully confirmed by the experiments of the team led by REED in which he took an active part.

FISHER'S EXACT TEST The test for association in a two-by-two table that is based upon the exact hypergeometric distribution of the frequencies within the table.

FISHING EXPEDITION Exploratory study to find clues and leads for further study. Although the term is sometimes used pejoratively, "fishing expeditions" may be done for worthwhile causes, e.g., to seek clues to the cause of a major life-threatening outbreak. A recent example was the initial investigation of Legionnaires' disease.

FITNESS This word has specific meanings in several fields related to epidemiology.
1. In population genetics, a measure of the relative survival and reproductive success of a given individual or phenotype, or population subgroup.
2. In health promotion, health risk appraisal, physical fitness is a set of attributes

that people have or achieve, that relate to their ability to perform physical activity. Intellectual and emotional fitness can also be described and to some extent measured.

FIXED COHORT A cohort in which membership is fixed by being present at some defining event ("zero time"); an example is the cohort comprising survivors of the atomic bomb exploded at Hiroshima. See also CLOSED COHORT.

FOLLOW-UP Observation over a period of time of an individual, group, or initially defined population whose appropriate characteristics have been assessed in order to observe changes in health status or health-related variables. See also COHORT.

FOLLOW-UP STUDY

1. A study in which individuals or populations, selected on the basis of whether they have been exposed to risk, received a specified preventive or therapeutic procedure, or possess a certain characteristic, are followed to assess the outcome of exposure, the procedure, or effect of the characteristic, e.g., occurrence of disease.

2. Synonym for COHORT STUDY.

FOMITES (singular, fomes) Articles that convey infection to others because they have been contaminated by pathogenic organisms. Examples include handkerchief, drinking glass, door handle, clothing, and toys.

FORCE OF MORBIDITY (Syn: hazard rate, instantaneous incidence density, instantaneous incidence rate, person-time incidence rate) Theoretical measure of the number of new cases that occur per unit of population-time, e.g., person-years at risk. This is a measure of the occurrence of disease at a point in time, t, defined mathematically as the limit, as Δt approaches zero, of

$$\frac{\text{Probability that a person well at time } t \text{ will develop} \atop \text{the disease in the interval } t + \Delta t}{\Delta t}$$

The average value of this quantity over the interval t to $(t + \Delta t)$ can be estimated as

$$\frac{\text{Incident cases observed from } t \text{ to } (t + \Delta t)}{\text{Number of person-time units of experience observed} \atop \text{from } t \text{ to } (t + \Delta t)}$$

FORCE OF MORTALITY (Syn: actuarial death rate) The hazard rate of the occurrence of death at a point in time t, i.e., the limit as Δt approaches zero, of the probability that an individual alive at time t will die by time $t + \Delta t$, divided by Δt. Distinct from cumulative death rate.

FORECASTING A method of estimating what may happen in the future that relies on extrapolation of existing trends (demographic, epidemiologic, etc.). It may be less useful than SCENARIO BUILDING, which has greater flexibility. For example, extrapolation of mortality trends for coronary heart disease in the early 1960s in the United States suggested that the mortality rates would continue to rise, perhaps indefinitely, whereas in fact the rates began to fall soon after that time.

FORTUITOUS RELATIONSHIP A relationship that occurs by chance and needs no further explanation.

FORWARD SURVIVAL ESTIMATE A procedure for estimating the age distribution at some later date by projecting forward an observed age distribution. The procedure uses survival ratios, often obtained from model life tables.

FOURFOLD TABLE See CONTINGENCY TABLE.

FRACASTORIUS, GIROLAMO (1484–1553) Physician, poet, natural scientist, and a man of legends, said to have required surgery at birth to open fused lips and to have survived a lightning bolt that killed his mother while he was in her arms as an infant. He gave the word "syphilis" to the world in his mock-heroic poem, *Syphilis Sive Morbus Gallicus* (1530), which explicitly described the transmission of disease by acts of venery. In *De Contagione* (1546), he described transmission of infection by direct contact, by fomites, and "at a distance," by which he meant droplets.

FRAMINGHAM STUDY Probably the best known cohort study of heart disease. Since 1949, samples of residents of Framingham, Massachusetts, have been subjects of investigations of risk factors in relation to the occurrence of heart disease and later, other outcomes.

FRANK, JOHANN PIETER (1745–1821) Author of *System einer vollständigen medicinischen Polizey,* which established hygiene as a systematic science and contained many suggestions based on epidemiologic observations. In modern terminology, Frank was "Director-general of public health" to the Hapsburg empire in eighteenth century Vienna. His *System* contained many sensible rules for individual good health, and detailed specifications for public health practice.

FREQUENCY See OCCURRENCE.

FREQUENCY DISTRIBUTION See DISTRIBUTION.

FREQUENCY MATCHING See MATCHING.

FREQUENCY POLYGON A graphic illustration of a distribution, made by joining a set of points, for each of which the abscissa is the midpoint of the class and the ordinate, or height, is the frequency.

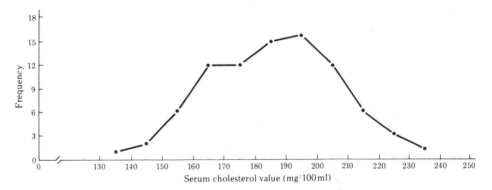

Frequency polygon. *From* Rimm et al., 1980.

FUNCTION A quality, trait, or fact that is so related to another as to be dependent upon and to vary with this other.

G

GALTON, FRANCIS (1822–1911) A founder of the modern science of human biology and the inventor of several statistical methods. Perhaps he is best known as the author of *Hereditary Genius* (1869), an analysis of physical and intellectual characteristics of successive generations of several hundred prominent families. Observing that off-spring of parents of unusual talent, height, etc., tended toward average, he formulated the "Law of filial regression" (the origin of the term "regression"). His statistical approaches were refined and extended by his pupil, KARL PEARSON, the founder of modern BIOMETRY.

GAUSSIAN DISTRIBUTION See NORMAL DISTRIBUTION.

GAME THEORY A branch of mathematical logic concerned with the range of possible reactions to a particular strategy; each reaction can be assigned a probability and each reaction can lead to further action by the "adversary" in the game. Used mainly in systems analysis and such applications as war-gaming, game theory has occasional applications in disease surveillance and control. It is also one of the underlying theories used in clinical decision analysis.

GENE A sequence of DNA that codes for a particular protein product or that regulates other genes. Genes are the biological basis of heredity and occupy precisely defined locations on chromosomes.

GENE POOL The total of all genes possessed by reproductive members of a population.

GENERAL FERTILITY RATE A more refined measure of fertility than the crude birth rate. The denominator is restricted to the number of women of childbearing age (i.e., 15–44 or 15–49). Defined as

$$\text{General fertility rate} = \frac{\text{Number of live births in an area during a year}}{\text{Midyear female population age 15–44 in same area in same year}} \times 1000$$

The upper age limit for this rate is 44 years in most jurisdictions.

GENERATION EFFECT (Syn: cohort effect) Variation in health status that arises from the different causal factors to which each birth cohort (see COHORT) in the population is exposed as the environment and society change. Each consecutive birth cohort is exposed to a unique environment that coincides with its life span.

GENERATION TIME The interval between receipt of infection by and maximal infectivity of the host. This applies to both clinical cases and inapparent infections.

With person-to-person transmission of infection, the interval between cases is determined by the generation time. See also INCUBATION PERIOD.

GENETIC DRIFT Random variation in gene frequency from generation to generation;

most often observed in small populations. The process of evolution through random statistical fluctuation of genetic composition of populations.

GENETIC EPIDEMIOLOGY The science that deals with the etiology, distribution and control of disease in groups of relatives, and with inherited causes of disease in populations.[1]

[1] Morton NE: *Outline of genetic epidemiology.* New York: Karger, 1982.

GENETIC LINKAGE Particular genes occupy specific sites in chromosomes, one member of each pair of chromosomes of course coming from each parent. When two genes are fairly close to each other in the same chromosome pair, they tend to be inherited together. Such genes are said to be linked, and the phenomenon is called genetic linkage.

GENETIC PENETRANCE The extent to which a genetically determined condition is expressed in an individual. This determines the frequency with which genetic effect is shown in a population.

GENETICS The branch of biology dealing with heredity and variation of individual members of a species. Its branches include population genetics, which overlaps epidemiology; therefore we include pertinent genetic terms in this dictionary.

GENOME The array of genes carried by an individual.

GEOGRAPHIC PATHOLOGY (Syn: medical geography) The comparative study of countries, or of regions within them, with regard to variations in morbidity/mortality. The (implied) aim of such study is usually to demonstrate that the variations are caused by or related to differences in the geographic environment.

GEOMETRIC MEAN See MEAN, GEOMETRIC.

GESTATIONAL AGE Strictly speaking, the gestational age of a fetus is the elapsed time since conception. However, as the moment when conception occurred is rarely known precisely, the duration of gestation is measured from the first day of the last normal menstrual period. Gestational age is expressed in completed days or completed weeks (e.g., events occurring 280–286 days after the onset of the last normal menstrual period are considered to have occurred at 40 weeks of gestation).

Measurements of fetal growth, as they represent continuous variables, are expressed in relation to a specific week of gestational age (e.g., the mean birth weight for 40 weeks is that obtained at 280–286 days of gestation on a weight-for-gestational-age curve). Some specified variations of gestational age are: *Preterm:* Less than 37 completed weeks (less than 259 days). *Term:* From 37 to less than 42 completed weeks (259–293 days). *Postterm:* Forty-two completed weeks or more (294 days or more).

"GOLD STANDARD" A jargon term, used to describe a method, procedure, or measurement that is widely accepted as being the best available. Often used to compare with new methods.

GOLDBERGER, JOSEPH (1874–1927) A U.S. Public Health Service physician. Responsible for a brilliant series of investigations of pellagra. After logical deductions led him to reject the prevailing view that pellagra had an infectious origin, he conducted studies in several rural communities and in institutions, leading conclusively to the demonstration that pellagra was a dietary deficiency disease.

GOMPERTZ'S LAW The proportionate relationship of mortality to age. Mortality is high during the first year of life (infancy), drops to its lowest level in childhood, and gradually climbs during the third and fourth decade. After age 35 or 40, the increase in mortality with age tends to be logarithmic for the remainder of the life span, i.e., the relative increase in mortality in each successive age class (of equal size) is about constant. This law was first enunciated by the demographer Benjamin Gompertz, on the basis of survival curves in English villages in the 1840s.

GONADOTROPHIC CYCLE One complete round of ovarian development in the mosquito (or other insect vector) from the time when the blood meal is taken to the time when the fully developed eggs are laid.

GOODNESS OF FIT Degree of agreement between an empirically observed distribution and a mathematical or theoretical distribution.

GOODNESS OF FIT TEST A statistical test of the hypothesis that data have been randomly sampled or generated from a population that follows a particular theoretical distribution or model. The most common such tests are chi-square tests.

GRADIENT OF INFECTION The variety of host responses to infection ranging from inapparent infection to fatal illness.

GRAPH Visual display of the relationship between variables; the values of one set of variables are plotted along the horizontal or x axis, of a second variable, along the vertical or y axis. Three-dimensional graphs of relationships between three variables can be represented and comprehended visually in two dimensions. The relationship between x and y may be linear, exponential, logarithmic, etc. See also AXIS, ABSCISSA, ORDINATE. "Graph" is also a descriptive term for histograms, bar charts, etc.

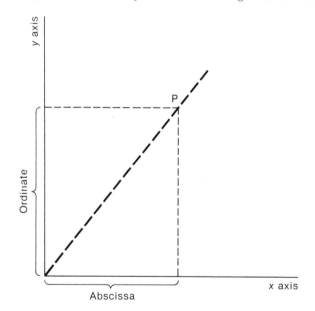

Graph showing abscissa, ordinate, and locus of a point, P,
in relation to x and y axis.

GRAUNT, JOHN (1620–1674) By profession a haberdasher, he was a member of the small community of scholars and natural scientists in London who were Fellows of the Royal Society in its early years and who made important contributions to the natural sciences. Graunt studied the BILLS OF MORTALITY and used them to conduct the first analytic studies of vital statistics, identifying differences in mortality rates between the sexes, between city and country folk, and recording all in *Natural and political observations mentioned in a following index and made upon the Bills of Mortality* (London, 1662).

GRAVIDITY The number of pregnancies (completed or incomplete) experienced by a woman.

GREENWOOD, MAJOR (1888–1949) Medical epidemiologist, trained in statistics by Karl Pearson; Greenwood was the first professor of epidemiology at the London School of Hygiene and Tropical Medicine. He inspired a whole generation of British epidemiologists, introducing to the subject a level of mathematical reasoning and statistical rigor it had not previously known. Author of many papers and several monographs, best known of which is *Epidemics and Crowd Diseases* (London, 1933).

GROSS REPRODUCTION RATE The average number of female children a woman would have if she survived to the end of her childbearing years and if, throughout that period, she were subject to a given set of age-specific fertility rates and a given sex ratio at birth. This rate provides a measure of replacement fertility in the absence of mortality. See also NET REPRODUCTION RATE.

GROWTH RATE OF POPULATION A measure of population growth (in the absence of migration) comprising addition of newborns to the population and subtraction of deaths. The result, known as *natural rate of increase,* is calculated as

$$\frac{\text{Live births during the year} - \text{deaths during the year}}{\text{Midyear population}} \times 100$$

Alternatively, it is the difference between crude birth rate and crude death rate.

H

HACKETT SPLEEN CLASSIFICATION A numerical means of recording the size of an enlarged spleen, especially in malaria. This is a 6-point scale of 0 (no enlargement) to 5 (enlarged to umbilicus or larger). See *Terminology of Malaria and of Malaria Eradication*. Geneva: WHO, 1963, pp. 40–41.

HALO EFFECT
1. The effect (usually beneficial) that the manner, attention, and caring of a provider have on a patient during a medical encounter regardless of what medical procedures or services the encounter involves. See also PLACEBO, PLACEBO EFFECT.
2. The influence upon an observation of the observer's perception of the characteristics of the individual observed (other than the characteristic under study) or the influence of the observer's recollection or knowledge of findings on a previous occasion.

HANDICAP Reduction in a person's capacity to fulfill a social role as a consequence of an IMPAIRMENT, inadequate training for the role, or other circumstances. Applied to children, the term usually refers to the presence of an impairment or other circumstance that is likely to interfere with normal growth and development or with the capacity to learn. See also INTERNATIONAL CLASSIFICATION OF IMPAIRMENTS, DISABILITIES, AND HANDICAPS for the official WHO definition.

HAPHAZARD SAMPLE Selection of a group of persons for study without thought as to whether they are representative of the population. The word "haphazard" here implies selection based on a mixture of criteria such as convenience, accessibility, turning up at the time an investigation or study is in progress, and belonging to some existing list or registry, etc. Because they have an unknown chance of being unrepresentative of the population, haphazard samples are unsatisfactory for generalization.

HARDY–WEINBERG LAW The principle that both gene and genotype frequencies will remain in equilibrium in an infinitely large population in the absence of mutation, migration, selection, and nonrandom mating. If p is the frequency of one allele and q is the frequency of another and $p+q=1$, then p^2 is the frequency of homozygotes for the allele, q^2 is the frequency of homozygotes for the other allele, and $2pq$ is the frequency of heterozygotes.

HARMONIC MEAN See MEAN, HARMONIC.

HAWTHORNE EFFECT The effect (usually positive or beneficial) of being under study upon the persons being studied; their knowledge of the study often influences their behavior. The name derives from work studies by Whitehead, Dickson, Roethlisberger, and others, in the Western Electric Plant, Hawthorne, Illinois, reported by Elton Mayo in *The Social Problems of an Industrial Civilization* (London: Routledge, 1949).

HAZARD A factor or exposure that may adversely affect health.

HAZARD RATE (Syn: force of morbidity, instantaneous incidence rate) A theoretical measure of the risk of occurrence of an event, e.g., death, new disease, at a point in time, t, defined mathematically as the limit, as Δt approaches zero, of the probability that an individual well at time t will experience the event by $t + \Delta t$, divided by Δt.

HEALTH The World Health Organization (WHO) described *health* in the preamble to its constitution as, "A state of complete physical, mental, and social well-being and not merely the absence of disease or infirmity." The WHO description of health has been criticized because of the difficulty of defining and measuring "complete" wellbeing.

There are several other definitions, including the following:

A state of dynamic balance in which an individual's or a group's capacity to cope with all the circumstances of living is at an optimum level.

A state characterized by anatomical, physiological and psychological integrity, ability to perform personally valued family, work and community roles; ability to deal with physical, biological, psychological and social stress; a feeling of well-being; and freedom from the risk of disease and untimely death.

Rene Dubos offered the following definition: "A modus vivendi enabling imperfect men to achieve a rewarding and not too painful existence while they cope with an imperfect world."

The word "health" is derived from the Old English *Hal,* meaning hale, whole, sound in wind and limb.

HEALTH BEHAVIOR The combination of knowledge, practices, and attitudes that together contribute to motivate the actions we take regarding health. Health behavior may promote and preserve good health, or if the behavior is harmful, e.g., tobacco smoking, may be a determinant of disease. This combination of knowledge, practices, and attitudes has been described and discussed by several writers, notably Becker.[1] See also *Illness behavior.*

[1] Becker MH (ed): *The Health Belief Model and Personal Health Behavior.* Thorofare NJ: Slack, 1974.

HEALTH CARE Those services provided to individuals or communities by agents of the health services or professions, for the purpose of promoting. maintaining, monitoring, or restoring health. Health care is broader than, and not limited to medical care, which implies therapeutic action by or under the supervision of a physician. The term is sometimes extended to include self-care.

HEALTH EDUCATION The process by which individuals and groups of people learn to behave in a manner conductive to the promotion, maintenance, or restoration of health.

HEALTH INDEX A numerical indication of the health of a given population derived from a specified composite formula. The components of the formula may be INFANT MORTALITY RATES, INCIDENCE RATES for particular disease, or other HEALTH INDICATORS.

HEALTH INDICATOR A variable, susceptible to direct measurement, that reflects the state of health of persons in a community. Examples include infant mortality rates, incidence rates based on notified cases of disease, disability days, etc. These measures may be used as components in the calculation of a HEALTH INDEX.

HEALTH PROMOTION The process of enabling people to increase control over and improve their health. It involves the population as a whole in the context of their everyday lives, rather than focusing on people at risk for specific diseases, and is directed toward action on the determinants or causes of health.

HEALTH RISK APPRAISAL (HRA) (Syn: health hazard appraisal [HHA]) A generic term applied to methods for describing an individual's chances of becoming ill or dying from selected causes. The many versions now available share several common features: Starting from the average risk of death for the individual's age and sex, a consideration of various lifestyle and physical factors indicates whether the individual is at greater or less than average risk of death from the commonest causes of death for his age and sex. All methods also indicate what reduction in risk could be achieved by altering any of the causal factors (such as cigarette smoking) that the individual could modify.

The premise underlying such methods is that information on the extent to which an individual's characteristics, habits, and health practices are influencing his future risk of dying will assist health care workers in counseling their patients.

HEALTH SERVICES Services that are performed by health care professionals, or by others under their direction, for the purpose of promoting, maintaining, or restoring health. In addition to personal health care, health services include measures for health protection and health education.

HEALTH SERVICES RESEARCH The integration of epidemiologic, sociological, economic, and other analytic sciences in the study of health services. Health services research is usually concerned with relationships between NEED, DEMAND, supply, use, and OUTCOME of health services. The aim of health services research is evaluation; several components of evaluative health services research are distinguished, viz:

Evaluation of *structure,* concerned with resources, facilities, and manpower.

Evaluation of *process,* concerned with matters such as where, by whom, and how health care is provided.

Evaluation of *output,* concerned with the amount and nature of health services provided.

Evaluation of *outcome,* concerned with the results, i.e., whether persons using health services experience measurable benefits such as improved survival or reduced disability.

HEALTH STATISTICS Aggregated data describing and enumerating attributes, events, behaviors, services, resources, outcomes, or costs related to health, disease, and health services. The data may be derived from survey instruments, medical records, and administrative documents. VITAL STATISTICS are a subset of health statistics.

HEALTH STATUS INDEX A set of measurements designed to detect short-term fluctuations in the health of members of a population; these measurements generally include physical function, emotional well-being, activities of daily living, feelings, etc. Most indexes require the use of carefully composed questions designed with reference to matters of fact rather than shades of opinion. The results are usually expressed by a numerical score that gives a profile of the well-being of the individual.

HEALTH SURVEY A survey designed to provide information on the health status of a population. It may be descriptive, exploratory, or explanatory. See also MORBIDITY SURVEY.

HEALTHY WORKER EFFECT A phenomenon observed initially in studies of occupational diseases: Workers usually exhibit lower overall death rates than the general population, due to the fact that the severely ill and disabled are ordinarily excluded from employment. Death rates in the general population may be inappropriate for comparison if this effect is not taken into account.

HEBDOMADAL MORTALITY RATE The mortality rate in the first week of life; the denominator is the number of live births in a year.

HENLE–KOCH POSTULATES See KOCH'S POSTULATES.

HERD IMMUNITY The immunity of a group or community. The resistance of a group to invasion and spread of an infectious agent, based on the resistance to infection of a high proportion of individual members of the group. The resistance is a product of the number susceptible and the probability that those who are susceptible will come into contact with an infected person. In the herd immunity equation, "probability of contact" is the intervening factor that reduces susceptibility to infection among group members to less than that anticipated from their susceptibility as unrelated individuals.

HETEROSCEDASTICITY Nonconstancy of the variance of a measure over the levels of the factors under study.

HIBERNATION See VECTOR-BORNE INFECTION.

HIPPOCRATES OF COS (c 460–370 BC) Greek physician, "Father of Medicine," responsible for careful clinical observation of many important and common diseases—tetanus, mumps, puerperal septicemia, etc. His writings contain important epidemiologic observations, as in the books *Airs, Waters, Places,* and *Epidemics.* His *Aphorisms* also demonstrate considerable empirical epidemiologic knowledge.

HISTOGRAM A graphic representation of the frequency distribution of a variable. Rectangles are drawn in such a way that their bases lie on a linear scale representing different intervals, and their heights are proportional to the frequencies of the values within each of the intervals. See also BAR DIAGRAM.

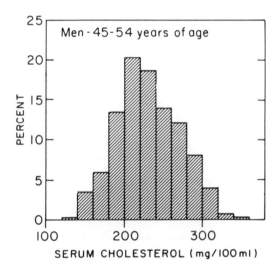

Histogram. *From* National Center for Health Statistics, 1978.

HISTORICAL COHORT STUDY (Syn: historical prospective study, nonconcurrent prospective study, prospective study in retrospect) A COHORT STUDY conducted by reconstructing data about persons at a time or times in the past. This method uses existing records about the health or other relevant aspects of a population as it was at some time in the past and determines the current (or subsequent) status of members of this population with respect to the condition of interest. Different levels of past exposure to risk factor(s) of interest must be identifiable for subsets of the population. See also COHORT STUDY.

HISTORICAL CONTROL Control subject(s) for whom data were collected at a time preceding that at which the data are gathered on the group being studied. Because of differences in exposures etc., use of historical controls can lead to bias in analysis.

HOGBEN NUMBER A unique personal identifying number constructed by using a sequence of digits for birthdate, sex, birthplace, and other identifiers. Suggested by the English mathematician Lancelot Hogben. Used in primary care epidemiology in some countries and usable in RECORD LINKAGE. See also IDENTIFICATION NUMBER; SOUNDEX CODE.

HOLMES, OLIVER WENDELL (1809–1894) Physician, poet, philosopher, autocrat ("of the Breakfast Table"), and crusader against puerperal fever. He argued that this was conveyed to patients by the contaminated hands and clothes of attending physicians and recommended washing the hands and changing clothes as a way to prevent it. Unlike SEMMELWEIS, he succeeded in convincing the medical profession. His correct belief was recorded in a paper, "The Contagiousness of Puerperal Fever."[1]

[1] *N Eng Q J Med Surg* 1:503–530, 1842–43.

HOLOENDEMIC DISEASE A disease for which a high prevalent level of infection begins early in life and affects most of the child population, leading to a state of equilibrium such that the adult population shows evidence of the disease much less commonly than do the children. Malaria in many communities is a holoendemic disease.

HOLOMIANTIC INFECTION See common source epidemic.

HOMOSCEDASTICITY Constancy of the variance of a measure over the levels of the factors under study.

HOSPITAL-ACQUIRED INFECTION See NOSOCOMIAL INFECTION.

HOSPITAL DISCHARGE ABSTRACT SYSTEM Abstraction of MINIMUM DATA SET from hospital charts for the purpose of producing summary statistics about hospitalized patients. Examples include the Hospital Inpatient Enquiry (HIPE) and Professional Activity Study (PAS). The statistical tabulations commonly include length of stay by final diagnosis, surgical operations, specified hospital service (i.e., medical, surgical, gynecological, etc.) and also give outcomes such as "death" and "discharged alive from hospital." This system cannot generally be used for epidemiologic purposes as it is not possible to infer representativeness or to generalize; this is because the data usually lack a defined denominator and the same person may be counted more than once in the event of two or more HOSPITAL SEPARATIONS in the period of study.

HOSPITAL INPATIENT ENQUIRY (HIPE) Statistical tables of a 10% sample of hospital patients in England and Wales, showing class of hospital, diagnosis, length of stay, outcomes, etc.

HOSPITAL SEPARATION A term used in commentaries on hospital statistics to describe the departure of a patient from hospital without distinguishing whether the patient departed alive or dead (the distinction is unimportant so far as the statistics of hospital activity such as bed occupancy are concerned).

HOST

1. A person or other living animal, including birds and arthropods, that affords subsistence or lodgment to an infectious agent under natural conditions. Some protozoa and helminths pass successive stages in alternate hosts of different species. Hosts in which the parasite attains maturity or passes its sexual stage are primary or definitive hosts; those in which the parasite is in a larval or asexual state are secondary or intermediate hosts. A transport host is a carrier in which the organism remains alive but does not undergo development.[1]

2. In an epidemiologic context, the host may be the population or group; biological, social, and behavioral characteristics of this group that are relevant to health are called "host factors."

[1] Benenson, *op. cit.*

HOUSEHOLD One or more persons who occupy a dwelling, i.e., a place that provides shelter, cooking, washing, and sleeping facilities; may or may not be a family. The term is also used to describe the dwelling unit in which the persons live.

HOUSEHOLD SAMPLE SURVEY A survey of persons in a sample of households. This, in many variations, is a favored method of gathering data for health-related and for many other purposes. The households may be sampled in any of several ways, e.g., by cluster, use of random numbers in relation to numbered dwelling units. The survey may be conducted by interview, telephone survey, or self-completed responses to present questions. The method is used in developing nations as well as in the industrial world.

HUMAN BLOOD INDEX Proportion of insect vectors found to contain human blood.

HUMAN ECOLOGY See ECOLOGY.

HUMAN IMMUNODEFICIENCY VIRUS (HIV) The pathogenic organism responsible for the acquired immunodeficiency syndrome (AIDS); formerly or also known as the lymphadenopathy virus (LAV), the name given by the original French discoverers Montagnier et al.[1] in 1983, or the human T-cell lymphotropic virus, type III (HTLV-III), the name given by Gallo et al.[2] to the virus they reported in 1984.

[1] Barre-Sinoussi F, Cherman JC, Rey F, et al.: Isolation of a T-lymphotropic retrovirus from a patient at risk for acquired immune deficiency syndrome (AIDS). *Science* 220:868–871, 1983.

[2] Gallo RC, Salahuddin SZ, Popovic M, et al.: Frequent detection and isolation of cytopathic retroviruses (HTLV-III) from patients with AIDS and at risk for AIDS. *Science* 224:500–503, 1984.

HYPERENDEMIC DISEASE A disease that is constantly present at a high incidence and/or prevalence rate and affects all age groups equally.

HYPERGEOMETRIC DISTRIBUTION The exact probability distribution of the frequencies in a two-by-two contingency table, conditional on the marginal frequencies being fixed at their observed levels.

HYPOTHESIS
1. A supposition, arrived at from observation or reflection, that leads to refutable predictions.
2. Any conjecture cast in a form that will allow it to be tested and refuted.
   See also NULL HYPOTHESIS.

I

IATROGENIC DISEASE Illness resulting from a physician's professional activity, or from the professional activity of other health professionals.

ICD See INTERNATIONAL CLASSIFICATION OF DISEASE.

ICEBERG PHENOMENON That portion of disease that remains unrecorded or undetected despite physicians' diagnostic endeavors and community disease surveillance procedures is referred to as the "submerged portion of the iceberg." Detected or diagnosed disease is the "tip of the iceberg." The submerged portion comprises disease not medically attended, medically attended but not accurately diagnosed, and diagnosed but not reported.[1]

[1] Last JM: The Iceberg. *Lancet,* 2:28–31, 1963.

ICHPPC See INTERNATIONAL CLASSIFICATION OF HEALTH PROBLEMS IN PRIMARY CARE.

IDENTIFICATION NUMBER, IDENTIFYING NUMBER Unique number given to every individual at birth or at some other milestone. Sweden has a system based on a sequence of digits for birthdate, sex, birthplace, and additional digits for each individual. Other systems, e.g., National Insurance number in the United Kingdom, Social Security number in the United States, and Social Insurance number in Canada, are sometimes used but are neither universal nor unique, being sometimes applied to whole families or at least to more than one individual. See also HOGBEN NUMBER; SOUNDEX CODE.

IDIOSYNCRASY Webster's Dictionary defines this as a distinctive characteristic or peculiarity of an individual. In pharmacoepidemiology, it means an abnormal reaction, sometimes genetically determined, following the administration of a medication.

ILLNESS See DISEASE.

ILLNESS BEHAVIOR Conduct of persons in response to abnormal body signals. Such behavior influences the manner in which a person monitors his body, defines and interprets his symptoms, takes remedial actions, and uses the health care system. See also HEALTH BEHAVIOR.

IMMUNITY, ACQUIRED Resistance acquired by a host as a result of previous exposure to a natural PATHOGEN or foreign substance for the host, e.g., immunity to measles resulting from a prior infection with measles virus.

IMMUNITY, ACTIVE Resistance developed in response to stimulus by an antigen (infecting agent or vaccine) and usually characterized by the presence of antibody produced by the host.

IMMUNITY, NATURAL Species-determined inherent resistance to a disease agent, e.g., resistance of man to virus of canine distemper.

IMMUNITY, PASSIVE Immunity conferred by an antibody produced in another host and acquired naturally by an infant from its mother or artificially by administration of an antibody-containing preparation (antiserum or immune globulin).

IMMUNITY, SPECIFIC A state of altered responsiveness to a specific substance acquired through immunization or natural infection. For certain diseases (e.g., measles, chickenpox) this protection generally lasts for the life of the individual.

IMMUNIZATION (Syn: vaccination) Protection of susceptible individuals from communicable disease by administration of a living modified agent (as in yellow fever), a suspension of killed organisms (as in whooping cough), or an inactivated toxin (as in tetanus). Temporary passive immunization can be produced by administration of antibody in the form of immune globulin in some conditions.

IMPAIRMENT A physical or mental defect at the level of a body system or organ. See also INTERNATIONAL CLASSIFICATION OF IMPAIRMENTS, DISABILITIES, and HANDICAPS for the official WHO definition.

INAPPARENT INFECTION (Syn: subclinical infection) The presence of infection in a host without occurrence of recognizable clinical signs or symptoms. Of epidemiologic significance because hosts so infected, though apparently well, may serve as silent or inapparent disseminators of the infectious agent. See also DISEASE, PRECLINICAL; DISEASE, SUBCLINICAL; VECTOR-BORNE INFECTION.

INCEPTION RATE The rate at which new spells of illness occur in a population; a term applied principally to short-term spells of illness such as acute respiratory infections, and preferred by some epidemiologists because an annual incidence rate for such conditions may exceed the numbers in the population at risk.

INCIDENCE (Syn: incident number) The number of instances of illness commencing, or of persons falling ill, during a given period in a specified population.[1] More generally, the number of new events, e.g., new cases of a disease in a defined population, within a specified period of time. The term incidence is sometimes used to denote INCIDENCE RATE.

[1] Prevalence and Incidence, *WHO Bul* 35:783–784, 1966.

INCIDENCE DENSITY The person-time incidence rate; sometimes used to describe the hazard rate. See FORCE OF MORBIDITY.

INCIDENCE-DENSITY RATIO (IDR) The ratio of two incidence densities. See also RATE RATIO.

INCIDENCE RATE The rate at which new events occur in a population. The numerator is the number of new events that occur in a defined period; the denominator is the population at risk of experiencing the event during this period, sometimes expressed as person-time. The incidence rate most often used in public health practice is calculated by the formula

$$\frac{\text{Number of new events in specified period}}{\begin{array}{c}\text{Number of persons exposed to risk}\\ \text{during this period}\end{array}} \times 10^n$$

In a dynamic population, the denominator is the average size of the population, often the estimated population at the mid-period. If the period is a year, this is the annual incidence rate. This rate is an estimate of the person-time incidence rate, i.e., the rate per 10^n person-years. If the rate is low, as with many chronic diseases, it is also a good estimate of the cumulative incidence rate. In follow-up studies with no censoring, the incidence rate is calculated by dividing the number of new cases in a specified period by the initial size of the cohort of persons being followed; this is equivalent to the cumulative incidence rate during the period. If the number of new cases during a specified period is divided by the sum of the person-time units at risk for all persons during the period, the result is the person-time incidence rate.

INCIDENCE STUDY See COHORT STUDY.

INCIDENT NUMBER See INCIDENCE.

INCUBATION PERIOD

1. The time interval between invasion by an infectious agent and appearance of the first sign or symptom of the disease in question.

2. In a VECTOR, the period between entry of the infectious agent into the vector and the time at which the vector becomes infective; i.e., transmission of the infectious agent from the vector to a fresh final host is possible (extrinsic incubation period).

INDEPENDENCE Two events are said to be independent if the occurrence of one is in no way predictable from the occurrence of the other. Two variables are said to be independent if the distribution of values of one is the same for all values of the other. Independence is the antonym of ASSOCIATION.

INDEPENDENT VARIABLE

1. The characteristic being observed or measured that is hypothesized to influence an event or manifestation (the dependent variable) within the defined area of relationships under study; that is, the independent variable is not influenced by the event or manifestation but may cause it or contribute to its variation.

2. In statistics, an independent variable is one of (perhaps) several variables that appear as arguments in a regression equation.

INDEX In epidemiology and related sciences, this word usually means a rating scale, e.g., a set of numbers derived from a series of observations of specified variables. Examples include the many varieties of health status index, scoring systems for severity or stage of cancer, heart murmurs, mental retardation, etc.

INDEX CASE The first case in a family or other defined group to come to the attention of the investigator. See also PROPOSITUS.

INDEX GROUP (Syn: index series)

1. In an experiment, the group receiving the experimental regimen.

2. In a case control study, the cases.

3. In a cohort study, the exposed group.

INDICATOR VARIABLE In statistics, a variable taking only one of two possible values, one (usually 1) indicating the presence of a condition, and the other (usually zero) indicating absence of the condition. Used mainly in REGRESSION ANALYSIS.

INDIRECT ADJUSTMENT See standardization.

INDIVIDUAL VARIATION Two types are distinguished:

1. *Intraindividual variation:* The variation of biological variables within the same individual, depending upon circumstances such as the phase of certain body rhythms and the presence or absence of emotional stress. These variables do not have a precise value, but rather a range. Examples include diurnal variation in body temperature, fluctuation of blood pressure, blood sugar, etc.

2. *Interindividual variation:* As used by Darwin, the term means variation *between* individuals. This is the preferred usage; the first usage is better described as personal variation.

INDUCTION PERIOD The period required for a specific cause to produce disease. More precisely, the interval from the causal action of a factor to the initiation of the disease. For example, a span of many years may pass between (presumably) radiation-induced mutations and the appearance of leukemia; this span would be the induction period for radiogenic leukemia. See also INCUBATION PERIOD; LATENT PERIOD.

INDUSTRIAL HYGIENE The science and art devoted to recognition, evaluation, and control of those environmental factors or stresses arising from or in the workplace, which may cause sickness, impaired health, and well-being, or significant discomfort and inefficiency among workers or among persons in the community. Alternatively, the profession that anticipates and controls unhealthy conditions of work to prevent illness among employees.

INFANT MORTALITY RATE (IMR) A measure of the yearly rate of deaths in children less than one year old. The denominator is the number of live births in the same year. Defined as

$$\text{Infant mortality rate} = \frac{\begin{array}{c}\text{Number of deaths in a year of}\\ \text{children less than 1 year of age}\end{array}}{\text{Number of live births in the same year}} \times 1000$$

This is often quoted as a useful indicator of the level of health in a community.

INFECTIBILITY The host characteristic or state in which the host is capable of being infected. See also INFECTIOUSNESS; INFECTIVITY.

INFECTION (Syn: colonization) The entry and development or multiplication of an infectious agent in the body of man or animals. Infection is not synonymous with infectious disease; the result may be inapparent or manifest. The presence of living infectious agents on exterior surfaces of the body is called "infestation" (e.g., pediculosis, scabies). The presence of living infectious agents upon articles of apparel or soiled articles is not infection, but represents CONTAMINATION of such articles. See also INAPPARENT INFECTION; TRANSMISSION OF INFECTION.

INFECTION, GRADIENT OF The range of manifestations of illness in the host reflecting the response to an infectious agent, which extends from death at one extreme to inapparent infection at the other. The frequency of these manifestations varies with the specific infectious disease. For example, human infection with the virus of rabies is almost invariably fatal, whereas a high proportion of persons infected in childhood with the virus of hepatitis A, experience a subclinical or mild clinical infection.

INFECTION, LATENT PERIOD OF The time between initiation of infection and first shedding or excretion of the agent.

INFECTION, SUBCLINICAL See INAPPARENT INFECTION.

INFECTIOUS DISEASE See COMMUNICABLE DISEASE.

INFECTIOUSNESS A characteristic of the disease that concerns the relative ease with which it is transmitted to other hosts. A droplet spread disease, for instance, is more infectious than one spread by direct contact. The characteristics of the portals of exit and entry are thus also determinants of infectiousness, as are the agent characteristics of ability to survive away from the host, and of infectivity.

INFECTIVITY
1. The characteristic of the disease agent that embodies capability to enter, survive, and multiply in the host. A measure of infectivity is the secondary attack rate.
2. The proportion of exposures, in defined circumstances, that results in infection.

INFERENCE The process of passing from observations and axioms to generalizations. In statistics, the development of generalization from sample data, usually with calculated degrees of uncertainty.

INFESTATION The development on (rather than in) the body of a pathogenic agent, e.g., body lice. Some authors use the term also to describe invasion of the gut by parasitic worms.

INFORMATION SYSTEM A combination of vital and health statistical data from multiple sources, used to derive information about the health needs, health resources, costs, use of health services, and outcomes of use by the population of a specified jurisdiction. The term may also describe the automatic release from computers of stored information in response to programmed stimuli. For example, parents can be notified when their children are due to receive booster doses of an immunizing agent against infectious disease.

INFORMED CONSENT Voluntary consent given by a subject or by a person responsible for a subject (e.g., a parent) for participation in an investigation, immunization program, treatment regimen, etc., after being informed of the purpose, methods, procedures, benefits, and risks. Awareness of risk is necessary for any subject to make an informed choice. The term also refers to consent for medical care.

INOCULATION See VACCINATION.

INPUT
1. The sum total of resources and energies purposefully engaged in order to intervene in the spontaneous operation of a system.
2. The basic resources required in terms of manpower, money, materials, and time.

INSTANTANEOUS INCIDENCE RATE See FORCE OF MORBIDITY.

INSTRUMENTAL ERROR Error due to faults arising in any or in all aspects of a measuring instrument, i.e., calibration, accuracy, precision, etc. Also applied to error arising from impure reagents, wrong dilutions, etc.

INTERACTION
1. The interdependent operation of two or more causes to produce or prevent an effect. *Biological interaction* means the interdependent operation of two or more causes to produce, prevent, or control disease. See also ANTAGONISM; SYNERGISM.
2. Differences in the effects of one or more factors according to the level of the remaining factor(s). See also EFFECT MODIFIER.
3. In statistics, the necessity for a product term in a linear model.

INTERMEDIATE VARIABLE (Syn: contingent variable, intervening [causal] variable, mediator variable) A variable that occurs in a causal pathway from an independent to a dependent variable. It causes variation in the dependent variable, and itself is caused to vary by the independent variable. Such a variable is statistically associated with both the independent and dependent variables.

INTERNAL VALIDITY See VALIDITY, STUDY.

INTERNATIONAL CLASSIFICATION OF DISEASE (ICD) The classification of specific conditions and groups of conditions determined by an internationally representative group of experts who advise the World Health Organization, which publishes the complete list in a periodically revised book, the *(Manual of the) International Statistical Classification of Diseases, Injuries and Causes of Death.* Every disease entity is assigned a number. There are 17 major divisions *(chapters)* and a hierarchical arrangement of subdivisions *(rubrics)* within each. Some chapters are "etiologic," e.g., Infective and Parasitic Conditions; more relate to body systems, e.g., Circulatory System; and some to classes of condition, e.g., neoplasms, injury (violence). The heterogeneity of categories reflects prevailing uncertainties about causes of disease (and classification in relation to causes). The Ninth Revision of the Manual (ICD-9) was published by WHO in 1977, after ratification in 1976.

INTERNATIONAL CLASSIFICATION OF HEALTH PROBLEMS IN PRIMARY CASE (ICHPPC) A classification of diseases, conditions, and other reasons for attendance for primary care. May be used for labeling conditions in problem-oriented records as used by primary care health workers. This classification is an adaptation of the ICD but makes more allowance for the diagnostic uncertainty that prevails in primary care. This classification is now in its second revision (ICHPPC-2). See also PROBLEM-ORIENTED MEDICAL RECORD.

INTERNATIONAL CLASSIFICATION OF IMPAIRMENTS, DISABILITIES, AND HANDICAPS (ICIDH) First published by WHO in 1980, this is an attempt to produce a systematic taxonomy of the consequences of injury and disease.

An *impairment* is defined in ICIDH as any loss or abnormality of psychological, physiological, or anatomical structure or function. It is concerned with abnormalities of body structure and appearance and with organ or system function resulting from any cause; in principle, impairments represent disturbances at the organ level.

A *disability* is defined in ICIDH as any restriction or lack (resulting from an impairment) of ability to perform an activity in a manner or within the range considered normal for a human being. The term disability reflects the consequences of impairment in terms of functional performance and activity by the individual; disabilities thus represent disturbances at the level of the person.

A *handicap* is defined in ICIDH as a disadvantage for a given individual, resulting from an impairment or a disability, that limits or prevents the fulfillment of a role that is normal (depending on age, sex, and social and cultural practice) for that individual. The term handicap thus reflects interaction with and adaptation to the individual's surroundings.

INTERNATIONAL COMPARISON See GEOGRAPHIC PATHOLOGY. See also CROSS-CULTURAL STUDY.

INTERNAL VALIDITY See VALIDITY, STUDY.

INTERPOLATE, INTERPOLATION To predict the value of variates within the range of observations; the resulting prediction.

INTERVAL INCIDENCE DENSITY See PERSON-TIME INCIDENCE RATE.

INTERVAL SCALE See MEASUREMENT SCALE.

INTERVENING CAUSE See INTERMEDIATE VARIABLE.

INTERVENING VARIABLE.
1. Synonym for INTERMEDIATE VARIABLE.
2. A variable whose value is altered in order to block or alter the effect(s) of another factor.

See also CAUSALITY, FACTORS IN.

INTERVENTION STUDY An epidemiologic investigation designed to test a hypothesized cause-effect relationship by modifying a supposed causal factor in a population.

INTERVIEW SCHEDULE The precisely designed set of questions used in an interview. See also SURVEY INSTRUMENT.

INVOLUNTARY SMOKING (Syn: passive smoking) The inhalation by nonsmokers of tobacco smoke left in the air by smokers; includes both smoke exhaled by smokers and smoke released directly from burning tobacco into ambient air; the latter is called sidestream smoke and contains higher proportions of toxic and other carcinogenic substances than exhaled smoke. The adjective "involuntary" is preferable to "passive" as the latter implies acquiescence—increasingly, nonsmokers are anything but acquiescent about this form of air pollution. "Passive" is, however, customary WHO usage.

ISLAND POPULATION A group of individuals isolated from larger groups and possessing a relatively limited gene pool; alternatively, a group that is immunologically isolated and may therefore be unduly susceptible to infection with alien pathogens.

ISOLATE (noun) Term used in genetics to describe a subpopulation (generally small) in which matings take place exclusively with other members of the same subpopulation.

ISOLATION

1. In microbiology, the separation of an organism from others, usually by making serial cultures.

2. Separation, for the period of communicability, of infected persons or animals from others in such places and under such conditions as to prevent or limit the direct or indirect transmission of the infectious agent from those infected to those who are susceptible or who may spread the agent to others. *Control of Communicable Disease in Man*[1] lists seven categories of isolation as follows:

    a. *Strict isolation:* This category is designed to prevent transmission of highly contagious or virulent infections that may be spread by both air and contact. The specifications, in addition to those above, include a private room and the use of masks, gowns, and gloves for all persons entering the room. Special ventilation requirements with the room at negative pressure to surrounding areas are desirable.

    b. *Contact isolation:* For less highly transmissible or serious infections, for diseases or conditions that are spread primarily by close or direct contact. In addition to the basic requirements, a private room is indicated but patients infected with the same pathogen may share a room. Masks are indicated for those who come close to the patient, gowns are indicated if soiling is likely, and gloves are indicated for touching infectious material.

    c. *Respiratory isolation:* To prevent transmission of infectious diseases over short distances through the air, a private room is indicated but patients infected with the same organism may share a room. In addition to the basic requirements, masks are indicated for those who come in close contact with the patient; gowns and gloves are not indicated.

    d. *Tuberculosis isolation (AFB isolation):* For patients with pulmonary tuberculosis who have a positive sputum smear or chest-x-rays that strongly suggest active tuberculosis. Specifications include use of a private room with special ventilation and the door closed. In addition to the basic requirements, masks are used only if the patient is coughing and does not reliably and consistently cover the mouth. Gowns are used to prevent gross contamination of clothing. Gloves are not indicated.

    e. *Enteric precautions:* For infections transmitted by direct or indirect contact with feces. In addition to the basic requirements, specifications include use of a private room if patient hygiene is poor. Masks are not indicated; gowns should be used if soiling is likely and gloves are to be used for touching contaminated materials.

    f. *Drainage/secretion precautions:* To prevent infections transmitted by direct or indirect contact with purulent material or drainage from an infected body site. A private room and masking are not indicated; in addition to the basic requirements, gowns should be used if soiling is likely and gloves used for touching contaminated materials.

g. *Blood/body fluid precautions:* To prevent infections that are transmitted by direct or indirect contact with infected blood or body fluids. In addition to the basic requirements, a private room is indicated if patient hygiene is poor; masks are not indicated; gowns should be used if soiling of clothing with blood or body fluids is likely. Gloves should be used for touching blood or body fluids.

See also QUARANTINE.

[1] Benenson AS (Ed): *Control of Communicable Diseases in Man,* 14th ed. Washington DC: American Public Health Association, 1985.

ISOMETRIC CHART A chart or graph that portrays three dimensions on a plane surface.

J, K

JACKKNIFE A technique for estimating the variance and the bias of an estimator. If the sample size is n, the estimator is applied to each subsample of size $n-1$, obtained by dropping a measurement from analysis. The sum of squared differences between each of the resulting estimates and their mean, multiplied by $(n-1)/n$, is the jackknife estimate of variance; the difference between the mean and the original estimate, multiplied by $(n-1)$, is the jackknife estimate of bias.

JENNER, EDWARD (1749–1823) An English physician and naturalist. On the basis of the observation that dairymaids who had had cowpox never got smallpox, he inoculated a boy age 10 with cowpox (vaccinia) in 1796. Over the succeeding two years he inoculated 22 more persons and then attempted to inoculate them with smallpox, always without inducing this infection. The results of his work were published in *An Inquiry into the Cause and Effects of the Variolae Vaccinae* (London, 1798). This successful method of immunizing persons and populations against smallpox led directly to the ultimate worldwide eradication of smallpox in 1977.

KAP (KNOWLEDGE, ATTITUDES, PRACTICE) SURVEY A formal survey, using face-to-face interviews, in which women are asked standardized pretested questions dealing with their knowledge of, attitudes toward, and use of contraceptive methods. Detailed reproductive histories and attitudes toward desired family size are also elicited. Analysis of responses provides much useful information on family planning and gives estimates of possible future trends in population structure. The term has sometimes been used to describe other varieties of survey of knowledge, attitudes, and practice, e.g., health promotion in general or in particular, cigarette smoking.

KAPPA A measure of the degree of nonrandom agreement between observers or measurements of the same categorical variable

$$k = \frac{P_0 - P_e}{1 - P_e}$$

where P_o is the proportion of times the measurements agree, and P_e is the proportion of times they can be expected to agree by chance alone. If the measurements agree more often than expected by chance, kappa is positive; if concordance is complete, kappa = 1; if there is no more nor less than chance concordance, kappa = 0; if the measurements disagree more than expected by chance, kappa is negative.

KENDALL'S TAU See CORRELATION COEFFICIENT.

KOCH, ROBERT (1843–1910) German physician, pathologist, and bacteriologist. One of the founders of microbiology and an important contributor to our understanding of infectious disease epidemiology. His major contributions to medical science include the life cycle of anthrax, the etiology of traumatic infection, methods of fixing and staining bacteria, and, in 1882, the discovery of the tubercle bacillus. The paper

70

reporting this contained the first statement of KOCH'S POSTULATES. In 1883, he discovered the cholera vibrio. He was awarded the Nobel Prize in 1905.

KOCH'S POSTULATES First formulated by Henle and adapted by Robert Koch in 1877, with elaborations in 1882. Koch stated that these postulates should be met before a causative relationship can be accepted between a particular bacterial parasite or disease agent and the disease in question.

1. The agent must be shown to be present in every case of the disease by isolation in pure culture.
2. The agent must not be found in cases of other disease.
3. Once isolated, the agent must be capable of reproducing the disease in experimental animals.
4. The agent must be recovered from the experimental disease produced.

See also CAUSALITY: EVANS'S POSTULATES.

KURTOSIS The extent to which a unimodal distribution is peaked.

L

LARGE SAMPLE METHOD (Syn: asymptotic method): Any statistical method based on an approximation to a normal or other distribution that becomes more accurate as sample size increases. An example is a chi square test on a set of frequencies.

LATENT IMMUNIZATION The process of developing immunity by a single or repeated inapparent asymptomatic infection. Not necessarily related to latent infection. See also IMMUNITY, ACQUIRED.

LATENT INFECTION Persistence of an infectious agent within the host without symptoms (and often without demonstrable presence in blood, tissues, or bodily secretions of host).

LATENT PERIOD (Syn: latency) Delay between exposure to a disease-causing agent and the appearance of manifestations of the disease. After exposure to ionizing radiation, for instance, there is a latent period of five years, on average, before development of leukemia, and more than 20 years before development of certain other malignant conditions. The term "latent period" is often used synonymously with "induction period," that is, the period between exposure to a disease-causing agent and the appearance of manifestations of the disease. It has also been defined as the period from disease initiation to disease detection. See also INCUBATION PERIOD; INDUCTION PERIOD.

LATIN SQUARE One of the basic statistical designs for experiments that aim at removing from the experimental error the variation from two sources, which may be identified with the rows and columns of the square. In such a design the allocation of k experimental treatments in the cells of a k by k (latin) square is such that each treatment occurs exactly once in each row and column. A design for a 5×5 square is as follows:

A	B	C	D	E
B	A	E	C	D
C	D	A	E	B
D	E	B	A	C
E	C	D	B	A

After Kendall and Buckland.[1]

[1] Kendall MG, Buckland AA: *A Dictionary of Statistical Terms*, 4th ed. London: Longman, 1982.

LAVERAN, ALPHONSE (1845–1922) French army surgeon who discovered the malaria parasite (1880) while on service in Algeria. Though initially sceptical, the scientific community soon accepted the validity of Laveran's discovery, which was confirmed and enlarged by Golgi, Grassi, and others. Laveran was awarded the Nobel Prize for medicine in 1907.

LEAD TIME The time gained in treating or controlling a disease when detection is earlier than usual, e.g., in the presymptomatic stage, as when screening procedures are used for detection.

LEAD TIME BIAS (Syn: zero time shift) Overestimation of survival time, due to the backward shift in the starting point for measuring survival that arises when diseases such as cancer are detected early, as by screening procedures.

LEAST SQUARES A principle of estimation, due to Gauss, in which the estimates of a set of parameters in a statistical model are those quantities that minimize the sum of squared differences between the observed values of the dependent variable and the values predicted by the model.

LEDERMANN FORMULA Ledermann[1] showed empirically that the frequency distribution of alcohol consumption in the population of consumers may be log-normal; the curve is sharply skewed—approximately one-third of drinkers consume more than 60% of the total amount of alcohol. Among drinkers the proportion of persons with alcoholism remains constant at around 7–9%. The pattern of consumption of illicit drugs among users may also be log-normal. Questions have been raised, however, about the validity of some assumptions upon which the formula is based.

[1] Ledermann S: *Alcool, Alcoolisme et Alcoolisation*. Paris: Presses universitaires de France, 1956.

LEEUWENHOEK, ANTONI VAN (1632–1723) An early microscopist from Delft, in the Netherlands, the first to use his microscopes to examine and describe small creatures *(animalcules)* such as the protozoan organisms in vaginal secretions, spermatozoa, and with growing ability to make more powerful microscopes, infectious microorganism. He was thus a key figure in the development of the germ theory of disease.

LEVIN'S ATTRIBUTABLE RISK See ATTRIBUTABLE FRACTION (POPULATION).

LIFE EVENTS Changes or disruptions in the pattern of living that may be associated with or produce changes in health. The relationship of "life stress" and "emotional stress" to onset of several kinds of serious chronic disease such as coronary heart disease and hypertension has been the subject of epidemiologic studies. The Rahe–Holmes Social Readjustment Rating Scale[1] was the first to be developed to assign ranks or ratings to significant life events such as death of a spouse or other close relative, loss of regular job, relocation, marriage, divorce, etc. Many other rating scales have since been developed.

[1] Holmes TH, Rahe RH: The social readjustment rating scale. *J Psychosomatic Res* 1:213–218, 1967.

LIFE EXPECTANCY See EXPECTATION OF LIFE.

LIFE EXPECTANCY FREE FROM DISABILITY (LEFD) An estimate of life expectancy adjusted for activity-limitation (data for which are derived from hospital discharge statistics, etc.). See also QALY.

LIFE STYLE The set of habits and customs that is influenced, modified, encouraged, or constrained by the lifelong process of socialization. These habits and customs include use of substances such as alcohol, tobacco, tea, coffee; dietary habits, exercise, etc., which have important implications for health and are often the subject of epidemiologic investigations.

LIFE TABLE A summarizing technique used to describe the pattern of mortality and survival in populations. The survival data are time specific and cumulative probabilities of survival of a group of individuals subject, throughout life, to the age-specific death rates in question. The life table method can be applied to the study not only of death, but also of any defined endpoint such as the onset of disease or the occurrence of specific complication(s) of disease. The survivors to age x are denoted by the symbol l_x, the expectation of life at age x is denoted by the symbol

$\mathring{e}_x$, and the proportion alive at age x who die between age x and $x+1$ years is denoted by the symbol nq_x. The life table method is used extensively in epidemiology and in many assessments of treatment regimens in clinical practice.

The first rudimentary life tables were published in 1693 by the astronomer Edmund Halley. These made use of records of the funerals in the city of Breslau. In 1815 in England, the first actuarially correct life table was published, based on both population and death data classified by age.

Two types of life tables may be distinguished according to the reference year of the table: the current or period life table and the generation or cohort life table.

The current life table is a summary of mortality experience over a brief period (one to three years), and the population data relate to the middle of that period (usually close to the date of a census). A current life table therefore represents the combined mortality experience by age of the population in a particular short period of time.

The cohort or generation life table describes the actual survival experience of a group, or cohort, of individuals born at about the same time. Theoretically, the mortality experience of the persons in the cohort would be observed from their moment of birth through each consecutive age in successive calendar years until all of them die.

The clinical life table describes the outcome experience of a group or cohort of individuals classified according to their exposure or treatment history.

Life tables are also classified according to the length of age interval in which the data are presented. A complete life table contains data for every single year of age from birth to the last applicable age. An abridged life table contains data by intervals of five or ten years of age. See also EXPECTATION OF LIFE: SURVIVORSHIP STUDY.

LIFE TABLE, EXPECTATION OF LIFE FUNCTION, $\mathring{e}_x$ (Syn: average future lifetime) The expectation of life function is a statement of the average number of years of life remaining to persons who survive to age x.

LIFE TABLE, SURVIVORSHIP FUNCTION, l_x The survivorship function is a statement of the number of persons out of an initial population of defined size, e.g., 100,000 live births, who would survive or remain free of a defined endpoint condition to age x under the age-specific rates for the specified year. The value of l_{40}, for example, is determined by the cumulative operation of the specific death rates for all ages below 40.

LIFETIME RISK The risk to an individual that a given health effect will occur at any time after exposure, without regard for the time at which that effect occurs.

LIKELIHOOD FUNCTION A function constructed from a statistical model and a set of observed data, which gives the probability of the observed data for various values of the unknown model parameters. The parameter values that maximize the probability are the maximum likelihood estimates of the parameters.

LIKELIHOOD RATIO TEST A statistical test based on the ratio of the maximum value of the likelihood function under one statistical model to the maximum value under another statistical model; the models differ in that one includes, the other excludes, one or more parameters.

LIND, JAMES (1716–1794) British naval surgeon; contributed to improved hygiene aboard ships. Conducted what amounted to epidemiologic experiments (albeit with small numbers) which established that scurvy could be prevented by fresh fruits such as lemons and oranges.

LINEAR MODEL A statistical model in which the value of a parameter for a given value of a factor, x, is assumed to be equal to $a + bx$, where a and b are constants.

LINEAR REGRESSION Regression analysis of data using linear models.

LINKAGE See GENETIC LINKAGE; RECORD LINKAGE.

LIVE BIRTH WHO definition adopted by Third World Health Assembly, 1950: Live birth is the complete expulsion or extraction from its mother of a product of conception, irrespective of the duration of the pregnancy, which, after such separation, breathes or shows any other evidence of life, such as beating of the heart, pulsation of the umbilical cord, or definite movement of voluntary muscles, whether or not the umbilical cord has been cut or the placenta is attached; each product of such a birth is considered live born.

In the *Report of WHO Expert Committee on Prevention of Perinatal Mortality and Morbidity (Technical Report Series* 457, 1970), it is noted that the above definition requires the inclusion as live births of very early and patently nonviable fetuses and that accordingly it is not strictly applied. The committee suggested, therefore, that WHO should introduce a viability criterion into the definition so that very immature fetuses surviving for very short periods were excluded, even though they showed one or more of the transitory signs of life.

LOCUS

1. The position of a point, as defined by the coordinates on a graph.
2. The position that a gene occupies on a chromosome.

LOD SCORE In genetics, the log odds ratio of observed to expected distribution of genetic markers.

LOGISTIC MODEL A statistical model of an individual's risk (probability of disease y) as a function of a risk factor x:

$$P(y|x) = \frac{1}{1 + e^{-\alpha - \beta r}}$$

where e is the (natural) exponential function. This model has a desirable range, 0 to 1, and other attractive statistical features. In the multiple logistic model, the term βx is replaced by a linear term involving several factors, e.g., $\beta_1 x_1 + \beta_2 x_2$ if there are two factors x_1 and x_2.

LOGIT (Syn: log-odds) The logarithm of the ratio of frequencies of two different categorical outcomes such as healthy versus sick.

LOGIT MODEL A linear model for the logit (natural log of the odds) of disease as a function of a quantitative factor X:

$$\text{Logit (disease given } X=x) = \alpha + \beta x$$

This model is mathematically equivalent to the LOGISTIC MODEL.

LOG-LINEAR MODEL A statistical model that uses an ANALYSIS OF VARIANCE type of approach for the modeling of frequency counts in contingency tables.

LOG-NORMAL DISTRIBUTION If a variable Y is such that $X = \log Y$ is normally distributed, it is said to have log-normal distribution. This is a SKEW DISTRIBUTION. See also NORMAL DISTRIBUTION.

LONGITUDINAL STUDY See COHORT STUDY.

LOUIS, PIERRE-CHARLES-ALEXANDRE (1787–1872) French physician and mathematician. One of the founders of medical statistics, his research on tuberculosis, which included dissection of 358 specimens and study of 1960 clinical cases, led to publication of *Recherches anatomicopathologiques sur la phthisie* (Paris, 1825). This work and others are marked by rigorous numerical precision and demonstration of similarities and differences based upon numerical distribution of data. The Lilienfelds[1] have pointed out that Louis greatly influenced the development of statistics as applied in biology and medicine; he either taught or otherwise directly influenced many European, British, and American workers, including William Farr, John Simon, William Augustus Guy, and William Budd in England, George Shattuck, Elisha Barnett, and Alonzo Clark in the United States, and Joseph Skoda in Hungary; those he influenced handed on these important concepts to their own pupils.

[1] Lilienfeld AM, Lilienfeld D: Threads of epidemiological history, in *Foundations of Epidemiology*, 2nd Ed. (New York: Oxford, 1980), pp. 23–45.

LOW BIRTH WEIGHT See BIRTH WEIGHT.

"LUMPING AND SPLITTING" Derisive term describing the propensity of epidemiologists to group related phenomena or to separate phenomena that hitherto have been grouped. Epidemiologists are sometimes called "lumpers and splitters."

M

MALARIA ENDEMICITY Certain terms used to describe the occurrence of malaria, based on enlarged spleen rates are categorized by WHO as follows:

1. Hypoendemic: Spleen rate in children 2–9 years <10%.
2. Mesoendemic: Spleen rate 11–50%.
3. Hyperendemic: Spleen rate in children over 50%, in adults usually over 25%.
4. Holoendemic: Spleen rate in children constantly over 75%, adult rate low.

MALARIA PERIODICITY Recurrence at regular intervals of symptoms; periodicity may be quotidian, tertian, or quartan, according to the interval between paroxysms:

1. Quartan: Recurring every third day, i.e., day 1, day 4, day 7, etc.
2. Quotidian: Recurring daily.
3. Tertian: Recurring every alternate day, i.e., day 1, day 3 etc.

MALARIA PATENT PERIOD Period during which parasites are present in peripheral blood.

MALARIA REPRODUCTION RATE Estimated number of malarial infections potentially distributed by the average nonimmune infected individual in a community where neither persons nor mosquitoes were previously infected.

MALARIA SURVEY Investigation in selected age-group samples in randomly selected localities to assess malaria endemicity; uses spleen and/or parasite rates as measure of endemicity.

MALTHUS, THOMAS ROBERT (1766–1834) An English clergyman and natural scientist who argued in *An Essay on the Principle of Population* (London, 1798) that populations increase in geometric progression while food supplies increase only in arithmetical progression, thus making famine inevitable. His work justifies his recognition as one of the founders of demography, even though events proved his predictions wrong (at least in the short term).

MANSON, PATRICK (1844–1922) Studied tropical diseases in China and made many contributions of fundamental importance, notably the transmission of filariasis by culicine mosquitoes, parts of the life cycle of schistosomes. He investigated and observed many other tropical parasitic diseases and founded the London School of (Hygiene and) Tropical Medicine in 1898.

MANTEL–HAENSZEL ESTIMATE, MANTEL–HAENSZEL ODDS RATIO Mantel and Haenszel[1] provided an adjusted ODDS RATIO as an estimate of relative risk that may be derived from grouped and matched sets of data. It is now known as the Mantel–Haenszel estimate, one of the few eponymous terms of modern epidemiology.

The statistic may be regarded as a type of weighted average of the individual odds ratios, derived from stratifying a sample into a series of strata that are internally homogeneous with respect to confounding factors.

The Mantel–Haenszel summarization method can also be extended to the summarization of rate ratios and rate differences from follow-up studies.

[1] Mantel N, Haenszel W: Statistical aspects of the analysis of data from retrospective studies of disease. *J Natl Cancer Inst* 22:719–748, 1959.

MANTEL–HAENSZEL TEST A summary CHI-SQUARE TEST developed by Mantel and Haenszel for stratified data and used when controlling for CONFOUNDING

MARGIN OF SAFETY An estimate of the ratio of the no-observed-effect level (NOEL) to the level accepted in regulations.

MARGINALS The row and column totals of a contingency table.

MARKOV PROCESS A stochastic process such that the conditional probability distribution for the state at any future instant, given the present state, is unaffected by any additional knowledge of the past history of the system.

MASKED STUDY See BLINDED STUDY.

MASKING Procedure(s) intended to keep participant(s) in a study from knowing some fact(s) or observation(s) that might bias or influence their actions or decisions regarding the study.

MATCHED CONTROLS See CONTROLS, MATCHED.

MATCHING The process of making a study group and a comparison group comparable with respect to extraneous factors. Several kinds of matching can be distinguished:

Caliper matching is the process of matching comparison group subjects to study group subjects within a specified distance for a continuous variable (e.g., matching age to within two years).

Frequency matching requires that the frequency distributions of the matched variable(s) be similar in study and comparison groups.

Category matching is the process of matching study and control group subjects in broad classes such as relatively wide age ranges or occupational groups.

Individual matching relies on identifying individual subjects for comparison, each resembling a study subject on the matched variable(s).

Pair matching is individual matching in which study and comparison subjects are paired.

MATERNAL MORTALITY (RATE) The risk of dying from causes associated with childbirth is measured by the maternal mortality rate. For this purpose the deaths used in the numerator are those arising during pregnancy or from puerperal causes, i.e., deaths occurring during and/or due to deliveries, complications of pregnancy, childbirth, and the puerperium. Women exposed to the risk of dying from puerperal causes are those who have been pregnant during the period. Their number being unknown, the number of life births is used as the conventional denominator for computing comparable maternal mortality rates. The formula is

$$
\begin{aligned}
\text{Annual maternal} \\
\text{mortality rate}
\end{aligned}
=
\frac{
\begin{aligned}
&\text{Number of deaths from puerperal} \\
&\text{causes in a given geographic area} \\
&\text{during a given year}
\end{aligned}
}{
\begin{aligned}
&\text{Number of live births that} \\
&\text{occurred among the population of} \\
&\text{the given geographic area during} \\
&\text{the same year}
\end{aligned}
}
\times 1000 \text{ (or } 100{,}000)
$$

There is variation in the duration of the postpartum period in which death may occur and be certified due to "puerperal causes," i.e., "maternal mortality." According to WHO, a maternal death is defined as the death of a woman while pregnant or within 42 days of termination of pregnancy, irrespective of the duration and the site of pregnancy, from any cause related to or aggravated by the pregnancy or its management but not from accidental or incidental causes.

Maternal deaths should be subdivided into two groups: (1) direct obstetric deaths, resulting from obstetric complications of the pregnant state, and (2) indirect obstetric deaths, resulting from preexisting disease or conditions not due to direct obstetric causes.

Although WHO defines maternal mortality as death during pregnancy or within 42 days of delivery, in some jurisdictions, a period as long as a year is used.

MATHEMATICAL MODEL A representation of a system, process, or relationship in mathematical form in which equations are used to simulate the behavior of the system or process under study. The model usually consists of two parts: the mathematical structure itself, e.g., Newton's inverse square law or Gauss's "normal" law, and the particular constants or parameters associated with them, such as Newton's gravitational constant or the Gaussian standard deviation.

A mathematical model is deterministic if the relations between the variables involved take on values not allowing for any play of chance. A model is said to be statistical, stochastic, or random, if random variation is allowed to enter the picture. See also MODEL.

MAXIMUM ALLOWABLE CONCENTRATION (MAC) See SAFETY STANDARDS.

MAXIMUM LIKELIHOOD ESTIMATE The value for an unknown parameter that maximizes the probability of obtaining exactly the data that were observed.

McNEMAR'S TEST A form of the CHI-SQUARE TEST for matched-pairs data. It is a special case of the MANTEL–HAENSZEL TEST.

MEAN, ARITHMETIC A MEASURE OF CENTRAL TENDENCY. Calculable only for positive values. It is calculated by taking the logarithms of the values, calculating their arithmetic mean, then converting back by taking the antilogarithm.

MEAN, HARMONIC A MEASURE OF CENTRAL TENDENCY computed by summing the reciprocals of all the individual values and dividing the resulting sum into the number of values.

MEASURE OF ASSOCIATION A quantity that expresses the strength of association between variables. Commonly used measures of association are differences between means, proportions or rates, the rate ratio, the odds ratio, and correlation and regression coefficients.

MEASUREMENT The procedure of applying a standard scale to a variable or to a set of values.

MEASUREMENT, PROBLEMS WITH TERMINOLOGY There is sometimes uncertainty about the terms used to describe the properties of measurement: accuracy, precision, validity, reliability, repeatability, and reproducibility. Accuracy and precision are often used synonymously, validity is defined variously, and reliability, repeatability, and reproducibility are frequently used interchangeable.

Etymologies are helpful in making a case for preferred usages, but they are not always decisive. *Accuracy* is from the Latin *cura,* care, and while this may be of interest to those in the health field, it does not illuminate the origins of the standard definition, that is, "conforming to a standard or a true value" (*OED*). Accuracy is distinguished from precision in this way: A measurement or statement can reflect or represent a true value without detail. A temperature reading of 98.6°F is accurate, but it is not precise if a more refined thermometer registers a temperature of 98.637°F.

Precision (from Latin *praecidere,* cut short) is the quality of being sharply defined through exact detail. A faulty measurement may be expressed precisely, but may not be accurate. Measurements should be both accurate and precise, but the two terms are not synonymous. Consistency or reliability describes the property of measurements or results that conform to themselves.

Reliability (Latin *religare*, to bind) is defined by the *OED* as a quality that is sound and dependable. Its epidemiologic usage is similar; a result or measurement is said to be reliable when it is stable, i.e., when repetition of an experiment or measurement gives the same results. The terms "repeatability" and "reproducibility" are synonymous (the *OED* defines each in terms of the other), but they do not refer to a quality of measurement, rather only to the action of performing something more than once. Thus, a way of discovering whether or not a measurement is reliable is to repeat or reproduce it. The terms "repeatability" and "reproducibility," formed from their respective verbs, are used inaccurately when they are substituted for "reliability," a noun that refers to the measuring procedure rather than the attribute being measured. However, in common usage, both repeatability and reproducibility refer to the capacity of a measuring procedure to produce the same result on each occasion in a series of procedures conducted under identical conditions.

Validity is used correctly when it agrees with the standard definition given by the *OED:* "sound and sufficient." If, in the epidemiologic sense, a test measures what it purports to measure (it is sufficient) then the test is said to be valid. See also ACCURACY; PRECISION; RELIABILITY; REPEATABILITY; VALIDITY.

MEASUREMENT SCALE The complete range of possible values for a measurement (e.g., the set of possible responses to a question, the physically possible range for a set of body weights). Measurement scales are sometimes classified into five major types, according to the quantitative character of the scale:

1. *Dichotomous scale:* One that arranges items into either of two mutually exclusive categories.
2. *Nominal scale:* Classification into unordered qualitative categories; e.g., race, religion, and country of birth as measurements of individual attributes are purely nominal scales, as there is no inherent order to their categories.
3. *Ordinal scale:* Classification into ordered qualitative categories, e.g., social class (I, II, III etc.), where the values have a distinct order, but their categories are qualitative in that there is no natural (numerical) distance between their possible values.
4. *Interval scale:* An (equal) interval involves assignment of values with a natural distance between them, so that a particular distance (interval) between two values in one region of the scale meaningfully represents the same distance between two values in another region of the scale. Examples include Celsius and Fahrenheit temperature, date of birth.
5. *Ratio scale:* A ratio is an interval scale with a true zero point, so that ratios between values are meaningfully defined. Examples are absolute temperature, weight, height, blood count, and income, as in each case it is meaningful to speak of one value as being so many times greater or less than another value.

MEASURES OF CENTRAL TENDENCY A general term for several characteristics of the distribution of a set of values or measurements around a value or values at or near the middle of the set. The principal measures of central tendency are the mean (average), median, and mode. (See entries under each.)

MECHANICAL TRANSMISSION See VECTOR-BORNE INFECTION.

MEDIAN A MEASURE OF CENTRAL TENDENCY. The simplest division of a set of measurements is into two parts—the lower and the upper half. The point on the scale that divides the group in this way is called the "median."

MEDIATOR (MEDIATING) VARIABLE See INTERMEDIATE VARIABLE.

MEDICAL AUDIT A health service evaluation procedure in which selected data from patients' charts are summarized in tables displaying such data as average length of stay or duration of an episode of care, the frequency of diagnostic and therapeutic procedures, and outcomes of care arranged by diagnostic category. These are often compared with predetermined norms.

MEDICAL CARE See HEALTH CARE.

MEDICAL RECORD A file of information relating to transaction(s) in personal health care. In addition to facts about a patient's illness, medical records nearly always contain other information. The full range of data in medical records includes the following:

1. Clinical, i.e., diagnosis, treatment, progress, etc.
2. Demographic, i.e., age, sex, birthplace, residence, etc.
3. Sociocultural, i.e., language, ethnic origin, religion, etc.
4. Sociological, i.e., family (next of kin), occupation, etc.
5. Economic, i.e., method of payment (fee-for service, indigent, etc.).
6. Administrative, i.e., site of care, provider, etc.
7. "Behavioral," e.g., record of broken appointment may indicate dissatisfaction with service provided.

MEDICAL STATISTICS See BIOSTATISTICS.

MENDEL'S LAWS Derived from the pioneering genetic studies of Gregor Mendel (1822–1884). Mendel's first law states that genes are particulate units that segregate; i.e., members of the same pair of genes are never present in the same gamete, but always separate and pass to different gametes. Mendel's second law states that genes assort independently; i.e., members of different pairs of genes move to gametes independently of one another.

META-ANALYSIS The process of using statistical methods to combine the results of different studies. In the biomedical sciences, the systematic, organized and structured evaluation of a problem of interest, using information (commonly in the form of statistical tables or other data) from a number of independent studies of the problem. A frequent application has been the pooling of results from a number of small randomized controlled trials, none in itself large enough to demonstrate statistically significant differences, but in aggregate, capable of so doing. Meta-analysis has a qualitative component, i.e., application of predetermined criteria of quality (e.g., completeness of data, absence of biases), and a quantitative component, i.e., integration of the numerical information. Meta-analysis includes aspects of an overview, and of pooling of data, but implies more than either of these processes. Meta-analysis carries the risk of several biases.

METHODOLOGY The scientific study of methods. Methodology should not be confused with methods. Sad to say, the word "methodology" is all too often used when the writer means "method."

MIASMA THEORY An explanation for the origin of epidemics, the "miasma theory" was implied by many ancient writers, and made explicit by Lancisi in *De noxiis paludum effluviis* (1717). It was based on the notion that when the air was of a "bad quality" (a state that was not precisely defined, but that was supposedly due to decaying organic matter), the persons breathing that air would become ill. Malaria ("bad air") is the classic example of a disease that was long attributed to miasmata. "Miasma" was believed to pass from cases to susceptibles in these diseases considered contagious.

MIGRANT STUDIES Studies taking advantage of migration to one country by those from other countries with different physical and biological environments, cultural background and/or genetic makeup, and different morbidity or mortality experience. Comparisons are made between the mortality or morbidity experience of the migrant groups with that of their current country of residence and/or their country of origin. Sometimes the experiences of a number of different groups who have migrated to the same country have been compared.

MILL'S CANONS In *A System of Logic* (1856), J.S. Mill devised logical strategies (canons) from which causal relationships may be inferred. Four in particular are pertinent to epidemiology: the methods of agreement, difference, residues, and concomitant variation.

Method of agreement (first canon): "If two or more instances of the phenomenon under investigation have only one circumstance in common, the circumstance in which alone all the instances agree, is the cause (or effect) of the given phenomenon."

Method of difference (second canon): "If an instance in which the phenomenon under investigation occurs, and an instance in which it does not occur, have every circumstance in common save one, that one occurring only in the former, the circumstance in which alone the two instances differ is the effect, or cause or a necessary part of the cause, of the phenomenon."

Method of residues (fourth canon): "Subduct from any phenomenon such part as is known by previous inductions to be the effect of certain antecedents, and the residue of the phenomenon is the effect of the remaining antecedents."

Method of concomitant variation (fifth canon): "Whatever phenomenon varies in any manner whether another phenomenon varies in some particular manner, is either a cause or an effect of that phenomenon, or is connected with it through some fact of causation."

MINIMUM DATA SET (Syn: uniform basic data set) A widely agreed upon and generally accepted set of terms and definitions constituting a core of data acquired for medical records and employed for developing statistics suitable for diverse types of analyses and users. Such sets have been developed for birth and death certificates, ambulatory care, hospital care, and long-term care. See also BIRTH CERTIFICATE; DEATH CERTIFICATE; HOSPITAL DISCHARGE ABSTRACT SYSTEM.

MISCLASSIFICATION The erroneous classification of an individual, a value, or an attribute into a category other than that to which it should be assigned. The probability of misclassification may be the same in all study groups (nondifferential misclassification) or may vary between groups (differential misclassification).

MOBILITY, GEOGRAPHIC Movement of persons from one country or region to another.

MOBILITY, SOCIAL Movement from one defined socioeconomic group to another, either upward or downward. Downward social mobility, which can be related to impaired health (e.g., alcoholism, schizophrenia, or mental retardation), is sometimes referred to as "social drift."

MODE One of the MEASURES OF CENTRAL TENDENCY. The most frequently occuring value in a set of observations.

MODEL
1. An abstract representation of the relationship between logical, analytical, or empirical components of a system. See also MATHEMATICAL MODEL.
2. A formalized expression of a theory or the causal situation that is regarded as having generated observed data.
3. (Animal) model: an experimental system that uses animals, because humans cannot be used for ethical or other reasons.
4. A small-scale simulation, e.g., by using an "average region" with characteristics resembling those of the whole country.

In epidemiology the use of models began with an effort to predict the onset and course of epidemics. In the second report of the Registrar-General of England and Wales (1840), WILLIAM FARR developed the beginnings of a predictive model for communicable disease epidemics. He had recognized regularities in the smallpox epidemics of the 1830s. By calculating frequency curves for these past outbreaks, he estimated the deaths to be expected. See also DEMONSTRATION MODEL; MATHEMATICAL MODEL; THEORETICAL EPIDEMIOLOGY.

MODERATOR VARIABLE (Syn: qualifier variable) In a study of a possible causal factor and an outcome, a moderator variable is a third variable exhibiting statistical interaction by virtue of its being antecedent or intermediate in the causal process under study. If it is antecedent, it is termed a conditional moderator variable or EFFECT MODIFIER; if it is intermediate, it is a contingent moderator variable. See also INTERACTION; INTERMEDIATE VARIABLE.

MONITORING

1. The performance and analysis of routine measurements, aimed at detecting changes in the environment or health status of populations. Not to be confused with SURVEILLANCE. To some, monitoring also implies intervention in the light of observed measurements.
2. Ongoing measurement of performance of a health service or a health professional, or of the extent to which patients comply with or adhere to advice from health professionals.
3. In management, the continuous oversight of the implementation of an activity that seeks to ensure that input deliveries, work schedules, targeted outputs, and other required actions are proceeding according to plan.

MONOTONIC SEQUENCE A sequence is said to be monotonic increasing if each value is greater than or equal to the previous one, and monotonic decreasing if each value is less than or equal to the previous one. If equality of values is excluded, we speak of a strictly (increasing or decreasing) monotonic sequence.

MONTE CARLO STUDY, TRIAL Complex relationships that are difficult to solve by mathematical analysis are sometimes studied by computer experiments that simulate and analyze a sequence of events, using random numbers. Such experiments are called Monte Carlo trials, or studies, in recognition of Monte Carlo as one of the gambling capitals of the world.

MORBIDITY Any departure, subjective or objective, from a state of physiological or psychological well-being. In this sense, *sickness, illness,* and *morbid condition* are similarly defined and synonymous (but see DISEASE).

The WHO Expert Committee on Health Statistics noted in its Sixth report (1959) that morbidity could be measured in terms of three units: (1) persons who were ill; (2) the illnesses (periods or spells of illness) that these persons experienced; and (3) the duration (days, weeks, etc.) of these illnesses. See also HEALTH INDEX; INCIDENCE RATE; NOTIFIABLE DISEASE; PREVALENCE RATE.

MORBIDITY RATE A term, preferably avoided, used indiscriminately to refer to incidence or prevalence rates of disease.

MORBIDITY SURVEY A method for estimating the prevalence and/or incidence of disease or diseases in a population. A morbidity survey is usually designed simply to ascertain the facts as to disease distribution, and not to test a hypothesis. See also CROSS-SECTIONAL STUDY; HEALTH SURVEY.

MORTALITY RATE See DEATH RATE.

MORTALITY STATISTICS Statistical tables compiled from the information contained in DEATH

CERTIFICATES. Most administrative jurisdictions in all nations produce tables of mortality statistics. These may be published at regular intervals; they usually show numbers of deaths and/or rates by age, sex, cause, and sometimes other variables.

MULTICOLLINEARITY In multiple regression analysis, a situation in which at least some of the independent variables are highly correlated with each other. Such a situation can result in inaccurate estimates of the parameters in the regression model.

MULTIFACTORIAL ETIOLOGY See MULTIPLE CAUSATION.

MULTINOMIAL DISTRIBUTION The probability distribution associated with the classification of each of a sample of individuals into one of several mutually exclusive and exhaustive categories. When the number of categories is two, the distribution is called binomial. See also BINOMIAL DISTRIBUTION.

MULTIPHASIC SCREENING See SCREENING.

MULTIPLE CAUSATION (Syn: multifactorial etiology) This term is used to refer to the concept that a given disease or other outcome may have more than one cause. A combination of causes or alternative combinations of causes may be required to produce the effect.

MULTIPLE LOGISTIC MODEL See LOGISTIC MODEL.

MULTIPLE RISK Where more than one risk factor for the development of a disease or other outcome is present, and their combined presence results in an increased risk, we speak of "multiple risk." The increased risk may be due to the additive effects of the risks associated with the separate risk factors, or to SYNERGISM.

MULTIPLICATIVE MODEL A model in which the joint effect of two or more causes is the product of their effects. For instance, if factor a multiplies risk by the amount a in the absence of factor b, and factor b multiplies risk by the amount b in the absence of factor a, the combined effect of factors a and b on risk is $a \times b$. See also ADDITIVE MODEL.

MULTISTAGE MODEL A mathematical model, mainly for carcinogenesis, based on the theory that a specific carcinogen may affect one of a number of stages in the development of cancer.

MULTIVARIATE ANALYSIS A set of techniques used when the variation in several variables has to be studied simultaneously. In statistics, any analytic method that allows the simultaneous study of two or more DEPENDENT VARIABLES.

MUTATION Heritable change in the genetic material not caused by genetic segregation or recombination, which is transmitted to daughter cells and succeeding generations, provided it is not a dominant lethal factor.

MUTATION RATE The frequency with which mutations occur per gene or per generation.

N

NATIONAL DEATH INDEX A computerized central registry of deaths in the United States, started in 1979 and operated by the U.S. National Center for Health Statistics, that facilitates mortality followup; cf. CANADIAN MORTALITY DATA BASE.

NATURAL EXPERIMENT A term probably derived from JOHN SNOW's account of his investigation of the practices of water supply companies in relation to the cholera epidemics in London in the 1850s. It refers to naturally occurring circumstances in which populations have different exposures to a supposed causal factor in a situation resembling an actual experiment in which persons would be assigned to groups.

John Snow was able to trace the London outbreaks of cholera in the 19th century to water impurity as a result of comparisons made between two water companies. It would have been unethical to expose "test subjects" to infection, but the situation at the time afforded him the opportunity to make observations of crucial importance.

> To turn this grand experiment to account, all that was required was to learn the supply of water to each individual house where a fatal attack of cholera might occur . . . I resolved to spare no exertion which might be necessary to ascertain the exact effect of the water supply on the progress of the epidemic, in the places where all the circumstances were so happily adapted for the inquiry . . . I had no reason to doubt the correctness of the conclusions I had drawn from the great number of facts already in my possession, but I felt that the circumstances of the cholera-poisoning passing down the sewers into a great river, and being distributed through miles of pipes, and yet producing its specific effects was a fact of so startling a nature, and of so vast importance to the community, that it could not be too rigidly examined or established on too firm a basis. (Snow, *On the Mode of Communication of Cholera.* 1855)

NATURAL HISTORY OF DISEASE The course of a disease from onset (inception) to resolution. Many diseases have certain well-defined stages that, taken all together, are referred to as the "natural history of the disease" in question. These stages are as follows:

1. Stage of pathological onset.
2. Presymptomatic stage: from onset to the first appearance of symptoms and/or signs. SCREENING tests may lead to earlier detection.
3. Clinically manifest disease, which may progress inexorably to a fatal termination, be subject to remissions and relapses, or regress spontaneously, leading to recovery.

Detection and intervention can alter the natural history of disease. The term has also been used to mean "descriptive epidemiology of disease."

NATURAL HISTORY STUDY A study, generally longitudinal, designed to yield information about the natural course of a disease or condition.

NATURAL RATE OF INCREASE (DECREASE) See GROWTH RATE OF POPULATION.

NEAREST NEIGHBOR METHOD A means of analyzing the spatial patterns of a free-living population. A term from veterinary epidemiology. Random sampling points are located throughout an area and the distance from each point to the nearest individual is measured; alternatively, individuals are selected at random and from each of these the distance to the nearest neighbor is measured.

NECESSARY AND SUFFICIENT CAUSE A causal factor whose presence is required for the occurrence of the effect and whose presence is always followed by the effect. See also ASSOCIATION; CAUSALITY.

NEEDS (Syn: health needs, perceived needs, professionally defined needs, unmet needs) This term has both a precise and an all-but-indefinable meaning in the context of public health. We speak of needs in precise numerical terms when we refer to specific indicators of disease or premature death that require intervention because their level is above that generally accepted in the society or community in question. For example, an infant mortality rate two or three times greater than the national average in a particular community is an indicator of unmet health needs of infants in that community (not to be confused with a need for more or better medical care). It should be clear that even in this seemingly precise usage there are implied value judgments. It must be explicitly stated that "needs" always reflect prevailing value judgments as well as the existing ability to control a particular public health problem. Thus, sputum-positive pulmonary tuberculosis was not recognized as a health need in 1850 but was by 1900 in the industrialized nations; the ill effects of cigarette smoking must now be universally acknowledge as a health need; and child abuse is increasingly regarded as a public health problem, to which we could apply the term "professionally defined need."
(See Vickers GR: What sets the goals of public health. *Lancet* 1:599, 1958.)

NEONATAL MORTALITY RATE
1. In VITAL STATISTICS, the number of deaths in infants under 28 days of age in a given period, usually a year, per 1000 live births in that period.
2. In obstetric and perinatal research the term "neonatal mortality rate" is often used to denote the cumulative MORTALITY RATE of live-born infants within 28 days of age.

NESTED CASE CONTROL STUDY A case control study in which cases and controls are drawn from the population in a cohort study. As some data are already available about both cases and controls, the effects of some potential confounding variables are reduced or eliminated.

NET MIGRATION The numerical difference between immigration and emigration.

NET MIGRATION RATE The net effect of immigration and emigration on an area's population expressed as an increase or decrease per 1000 population of the area in a given year.

NET REPRODUCTION RATE The average number of female children born per woman in a cohort subject to a given set of age-specific fertility rates, a given set of age-specific mortality rates, and a given sex ratio at birth. This rate measures replacement fertility under given conditions of fertility and mortality: it is the ratio of daughters to mothers assuming continuation of the specified conditions of fertility and mortality. It is a measure of population growth from one generation to another under constant conditions. This rate is similar to the gross reproduction rate, but takes into account that some women will die before completing their childbearing years. An NRR of 1.00 means that each generation of mothers is having exactly enough daughters to replace itself in the population. See also GROSS REPRODUCTION RATE.

NEW YORK STATE IDENTIFICATION AND INTELLIGENCE SYSTEM (NYSIIS) A method of identifying individuals for RECORD LINKAGE based on phonetic spelling of full names, sequence of digits for birthdate, birthplace, sex, name at birth, and parents' names. See also HOGBEN NUMBER; SOUNDEX CODE.

NIDUS A focus of infection. The term can be used to describe any heterogeneity in the distribution of a disease, but is usually applied to a small area in which conditions

favor occurrence and spread of a communicable disease; also, the site of origin of
a pathological process.

NIGHTINGALE, FLORENCE (1820–1910) An English woman who is identified as the founder
of modern nursing, but was much more. In addition to her famous work of elevat-
ing nursing to a noble profession during the Crimean War, and establishing a training school for nurses at St. Thomas's Hospital in London, she recognized the importance of statistical analysis of hospital records (*Notes on Hospitals* London:
Longmans, 1859); her contributions were recognized by election to Fellowship of
the Royal Statistical Society. Her best-known work is *Notes on Nursing* (1860).

NOISE (IN DATA) This term is used when extraneous uncontrolled variables and/or errors influence the distribution of measurements that are made in a study, thus
rendering difficult or impossible the determination of relationships between variables under scrutiny.

NOMENCLATURE A list of all approved terms for describing and recording observations.

NOMINAL SCALE See MEASUREMENT SCALE.

NOMOGRAM A form of line chart showing scales for the variables involved in a particular
formula in such a way that corresponding values for each variable lie on a straight
line intersecting all the scales.

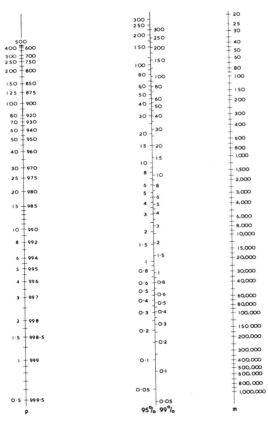

Nomogram of confidence limits to a rate.
From Rosenbaum, Nomograms for rates per 1000, *Br Med J* 1:169–170, 1963.

NONCONCURRENT STUDY See HISTORICAL COHORT STUDY.

NONDIFFERENTIAL MISCLASSIFICATION See MISCLASSIFICATION.

NONEXPERIMENTAL STUDY See OBSERVATIONAL STUDY.

NONPARAMETRIC METHODS See DISTRIBUTION-FREE METHOD.

NONPARAMETRIC TEST See DISTRIBUTION-FREE METHOD.

NONPARTICIPANTS (Syn: nonresponders) Members of a study sample or population who do not take part in the study for whatever reason, or members of a target population who do not participate in an activity. Differences between participants and nonparticipants have been demonstrated repeatedly in studies of many kinds, and this is often a source of BIAS.

NO-OBSERVED-EFFECT LEVEL (NOEL) A term from toxicology, meaning the highest dose at which no adverse health effects are detected in an animal population. A NOEL-SF is a no-observed-effects level with an added safety factor for human exposures, used in setting human safety standards.

NORM This term has two quite distinct meanings:
  1. The first is "what is usual," e.g., the range into which blood pressure values usually fall in a population group, the dietary or infant feeding practices that are usual in a given culture, or the way that a given illness is usually treated in a given health care system.
  2. The second sense is "what is desirable," e.g., the range of blood pressures that a given authority regards as being indicative of present good health or as predisposing to future good health, the dietary or infant feeding practices that are valued in a given culture, or the health care procedures or facilities for health care that a given authority regards as desirable.

  In the latter sense, norms may be used as criteria when evaluating health care, in order to determine the degree of conformity with what is desirable, the average length of stay of patients in hospital, etc. A distinction is sometimes made between norms, defined as quantitative indexes based on research, and standards, which are fixed arbitrarily.

NORMAL This term has three distinct meanings. Conceptual difficulties may arise if these different meanings are not specified, or if the area of their overlap is not clearly understood.
  1. Within the usual range of variation in a given population or population group; or frequently occurring in a given population or group. In this sense, "normal" is frequently defined as, "within a range extending from two standard deviations below the mean to two standard deviations above the mean," or "between specified (e.g., the 10th and 90th) percentiles of the distribution."
  2. In good health, indicative or predictive of good health, or conducive to good health. For a diagnostic or screening test, a "normal" result is one in a range within which the probability of a specific disease is low (see also NORMAL LIMITS).
  3. (Of a distribution) Gaussian; see also NORMAL DISTRIBUTION.

NORMAL DISTRIBUTION (Syn: Gaussian distribution) The continuous frequency distribution of infinite range represented by the equation

$$f(x) = \frac{1}{(2\pi\sigma^2)^{1/2}} e^{-(x-\mu)^2/2\sigma^2}$$

where x is the abscissa, $f(x)$ is the ordinate, μ is the mean, l is the natural logarithm, 2.718 and σ the standard deviation.

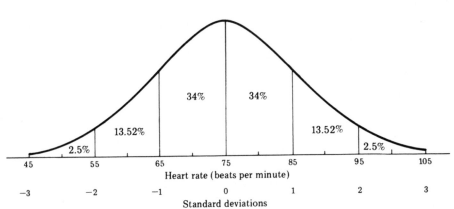

Normal distribution of heart rate. *From* Rimm et al., 1980.

The properties of a normal distribution include the following: (1) It is a continuous, symmetrical distribution; both tails extend to infinity; (2) the arithmetic mean,
mode, and median are identical; and (3) its shape is completely determined by the
mean and standard deviation.

NORMAL LIMITS The limits of the "normal" range of a test or measurement, in the sense
of being indicative of or conducive to good health. One way to determine normal
limits is to compare the values obtained when the measurements are made in two
groups, one that is healthy and has been found to remain healthy, the other ill, or
subsequently found to become ill. The result may be two overlapping distributions,
as illustrated. Outside the area where the distributions overlap, a given value clearly
identifies the presence or absence of disease or some other manifestation of poor
health. If a value falls into the area of overlap, the individual may belong to either
the normal or the abnormal group. The choice of the normal limits depends upon
the relative importance attached to the identification of individuals as healthy or
unhealthy. See also FALSE NEGATIVE; FALSE POSITIVE; SENSITIVITY AND SPECIFICITY.

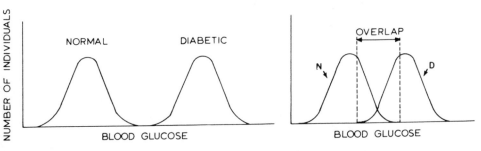

Hypothetical distribution of normal and diabetic glucose levels.
From Lilienfeld and Lilienfeld, 1979.

NORMATIVE Pertaining to the normal, usual, accepted standard or values. See also NORM.
NOSOCOMIAL Arising while a patient is in a hospital or as a result of being in a hospital;
relating to a hospital; denoting a new disorder (unrelated to the patient's primary
condition) associated with being in a hospital.

NOSOCOMIAL INFECTION (Syn: hospital-acquired infection) An infection originating in a medical facility, e.g., occurring in a patient in a hospital or other health care facility in whom the infection was not present or incubating at the time of admission. Includes infections acquired in the hospital but appearing after discharge; it also includes such infections among staff.

NOSOGRAPHY, NOSOLOGY Classification of ill persons into groups, whatever the criteria for their classification, and agreement as to the boundaries of the groups, is called "nosology." The assignment of names to each disease entity in the group results in a nomenclature of disease entities, or nosography. (Faber K: *Nosography in Modern Internal Medicine.* New York: Hoeber, 1923.)

NOTIFIABLE DISEASE A disease that, by statutory requirements, must be reported to the public health authority in the pertinent jurisdiction when the diagnosis is made.

A disease deemed of sufficient importance to the public health to require that its occurrence be reported to health authorities.

The reporting to public health authorities of communicable diseases is, unfortunately, very incomplete. The reasons for this include diagnostic inexactitude; the desire of patients and physicians to conceal the occurrence of conditions carrying a social stigma, e.g., sexually transmitted diseases; and the indifference of physicians to the usefulness of information about such diseases as hepatitis, influenza, and measles. Yet notifications are extremely important. They provide the starting point for investigations into the failure of preventive measures such as immunizations, for tracing sources of infection, for finding common vehicles of infection, for describing the geographic clustering of infection, and for various other purposes, depending upon the particular disease.

N.S., n.s. Abbreviation, usually written lower case, for not statistically significant.

NULL HYPOTHESIS (Syn: test hypothesis) The statistical hypothesis that one variable has no association with another variable or set of variables, or that two or more population distributions do not differ from one another. In simplest terms, the null hypothesis states that the results observed in a study, experiment, or test are no different from what might have occurred as a result of the operation of chance alone.

NUMERATOR The upper portion of a fraction used to calculate a rate or a ratio.

NUMERICAL TAXONOMY The construction of homogeneous groupings or taxa using numerical methods; allied to CLUSTER ANALYSIS.

O

OBSERVATIONAL STUDY (Syn: nonexperimental study, survey) Epidemiologic study in situations where nature is allowed to take its course; changes or differences in one characteristic are studied in relation to changes or differences in other(s), without the intervention of the investigator.

OBSERVER VARIATION (ERROR) Variation (or error) due to failure of the observer to measure or to identify a phenomenon accurately. Observer variation erodes scientific credibility whenever it appears. Sir Thomas Browne in *Pseudodoxia Epidemica* (1646), subtitled "Enquiries into very many commonly received tenents and presumed truths," recognized several sources of error: "the common infirmity of human nature, the erroneous disposition of the people, misapprehension, fallacy or false deduction, credulity, obstinate adherence to authority, the belief in popular conceits, the endeavours of Satan."

All observations are subject to variation. Discrepancies between repeated observations by the same observer and between different observers are to be expected; these can be diminished but probably never absolutely eliminated.

Variation may arise from several sources. The observer may miss an abnormality or think he has found one where none is present; a measurement or a test may give incorrect results due to faulty technique or incorrect reading and recording of the results; or the observer may misinterpret the information. Two varieties of observer variation are interobserver variation, i.e., the amount observers vary from one another when reporting on the same material, and intraobserver variation, the amount one observer varies between observations when he reports more than once on the same material.

OCCAM'S RAZOR (Syn: scientific parsimony) William of Occam's 14th century dictum was that, "the assumptions introduced to explain a thing must not be multiplied beyond necessity." This useful maxim does not contradict the conclusion that multiple causes operate in any system. The number of causes implicated depends on the frame of reference of the investigator and on the scope of the inquiry.

OCCURRENCE (Syn: frequency) In epidemiology, a general term describing the frequency of a disease or other attribute or event in a population without distinguishing between INCIDENCE and PREVALENCE.

ODDS The ratio of the probability of occurrence of an event to that of nonoccurrence, or the ratio of the probability that something is so, to the probability that it is not so. If 60 smokers develop a chronic cough and 40 do not, the odds among these 100 smokers in favor of developing a cough are 60:40, or 1.5; this may be contrasted with the probability that these smokers will develop a cough, which is 60/100 or 0.6.

ODDS RATIO (Syn: cross-product ratio, relative odds) The ratio of two odds. The term "odds" is defined differently according to the situation under discussion. Consider the following notation for the distribution of a binary exposure and a disease in a population or a sample.

	Exposed	Unexposed
Disease	*a*	*b*
No disease	*c*	*d*

The odds ratio (cross-product ratio) is *ad/bc*.

The *exposure-odds ratio* for a set of case control data is the ratio of the odds in favor of exposure among the cases *(a/b)* to the odds in favor of exposure among noncases *(c/d)*. This reduces to *ad/bc*. With incident cases, unbiased subject selection, and a "rare" disease (say, under 2% cumulative incidence rate over the study period), *ad/bc* is an approximate estimate of the RISK RATIO. With incident cases, unbiased subject selection, and DENSITY SAMPLING of controls *ad/bc* is an estimate of the ratio of the person-time incidence rates (FORCES OF MORBIDITY) in the exposed and unexposed (no rarity assumption is required for this).

The *disease-odds (rate-odds) ratio* for a cohort or cross section is the ratio of the odds in favor of disease among the exposed *(a/c)* to the odds in favor of disease among the unexposed *b/d)*. This reduces to *ad/bc* and hence is equal to the exposure-odds ratio for the cohort or cross section.

The *prevalence-odds ratio* refers to an odds ratio derived cross sectionally, as, for example, an odds ratio derived from studies of prevalent (rather than incident) cases.

The *risk-odds ratio* is the ratio of the odds in favor of getting disease, if exposed, to the odds in favor of getting disease if not exposed. The odds ratio derived from a cohort study is an estimate of this. See also CASE CONTROL STUDY.

ONE-TAIL TEST A statistical significance test based on the assumption that the data have only one possible direction of variability.

OPERATIONAL RESEARCH The systematic study, by observation and experiment, of the working of a system, e.g., health services, with a view to improvement.

OPERATIONS RESEARCH

1. The fitting of models to data, or the designing of models.
2. Synonym for OPERATIONAL RESEARCH.

OPPORTUNISTIC INFECTION Infection with organism(s) that are normally innocuous, e.g., commensals in the human, but become pathogenic when the body's immunologic defenses are compromised, as happens in the acquired immunodeficiency syndrome (AIDS).

ORDINAL SCALE See MEASUREMENT SCALE.

ORDINATE The distance of a point, *P*, from the horizontal or *x* axis of a graph, measured along the vertical or *y* axis. See also ABSCISSA; GRAPH.

OUTCOMES All the possible results that may stem from exposure to a causal factor, or from preventive or therapeutic interventions; all identified changes in health status arising as a consequence of the handling of a health problem. See also CAUSALITY; CAUSATION OF DISEASE, FACTORS IN.

OUTLIERS Observations differing so widely from the rest of the data as to lead one to suspect that a gross error may have been committed, or suggesting that these values come from a different population.

OUTBREAK (Syn: epidemic) Sometimes the preferred word, as it may escape sensationalism associated with the word epidemic. Alternatively, a localized as opposed to generalized epidemic.

OUTPUT The immediate result of professional or institutional health care activities, usually expressed as units of service, e.g., patient hospital days, outpatient visits, laboratory tests performed.

OVERMATCHING A situation that may arise when groups are matched. Several varieties can be distinguished:

1. The matching procedure partially or completely obscures evidence of a true causal association between the independent and dependent variables. Overmatching may occur if the matching variable is involved in, or is closely connected with, the mechanism whereby the independent variable affects the dependent variable. The matching variable may be an intermediate cause in the causal chain or it may be strongly affected by, or a consequence of, such an intermediate cause.

2. The matching procedure uses one or more unnecessary matching variables, e.g., variables that have no causal effect or influence on the dependent variable, and hence cannot confound the relationship between the independent and dependent variables.

3. The matching process is unduly elaborate, involving the use of numerous matching variables and/or insisting on very close similarity with respect to specific matching variables. This leads to difficulty in finding suitable controls.

See also MATCHING.

OVERWINTERING See VECTOR-BORNE INFECTION.

P

P, P (PROBABILITY) VALUE The probability that a test statistic would be as extreme as or more extreme than observed if the null hypothesis were true. The letter P, followed by the abbreviation n.s. (not significant) or by the symbol < (less than) and a decimal notation such as 0.01, 0.05, is a statement of the probability that the difference observed could have occurred by chance, if the groups are really alike, i.e., under the NULL HYPOTHESIS.

Investigators may arbitrarily set their own significance levels, but in most biomedical and epidemiologic work, a study result whose probability value is less than 5% ($P<0.05$) or 1% ($P<0.01$) is considered sufficiently unlikely to have occurred by chance to justify the designation "statistically significant." See also STATISTICAL SIGNIFICANCE.

PAIRED SAMPLES In a CLINICAL TRIAL, pairs of subject patients may be studied. One member of each pair receives the experimental regimen, and the other receives a suitably designated control regimen. Pairing should be based on a prognostic variable such as age

Pairing may similarly be used in a CASE CONTROL STUDY or in a COHORT STUDY. See also MATCHING.

PANDEMIC An epidemic occurring over a very wide area and usually affecting a large proportion of the population.

PANEL STUDY A combination of cross-sectional and cohort methods, in which the investigator conducts a series of cross-sectional studies of the same individuals or study sample. This method of study permits changes in one variable to be related to changes in other variables. See also NESTED CASE-CONTROL STUDY.

PANUM, PETER LUDWIG (1820–1885) A Danish physician who observed firsthand an epidemic of measles in the Faroe Islands in 1846. This was the first outbreak there for many years, and from the epidemic pattern, Panum deduced some basic, previously unknown details about the method of spread, and incubation period, the lasting immunity that followed infection, and the relationship between age and severity of infection.

PARADIGM A typical example, a pattern of thought or conceptualization; an overall way of regarding phenomena, within which scientists normally work. A paradigm may dictate what form of explanation will be found acceptable, but a science may change paradigms. In many contexts in which it is used, the term is both ambiguous and vague.[1] The word is often used loosely as a synonym for "factor" or "variable."

[1] Kuhn T. *The Structure of Scientific Revolutions.* Chicago: University of Chicago Press, 1962.

PARAMETER In mathematics, a constant in a formula or model; in statistics and epidemiology, a measureable characteristic of a population.

PARAMETRIC TEST A statistical test that depends upon assumption(s) about the distribution of the data, e.g., that these are normally distributed.

PARASITE An animal or vegetable organism that lives on or in another and derives its nourishment therefrom. An obligate parasite is one that cannot lead an independent nonparasitic existence. A facultative parasite is one that is capable of either parasitic or independent existence.

PARASITE COUNT See WORM COUNT.

PARASITE DENSITY The collective degree of parasitemia in a population, calculated by the use of either the geometric mean or the weighted average of the individual parasite counts; e.g., by using a frequency distribution based on a geometric progression.

PARATENIC HOST (Syn: transport host) A second, third, or subsequent intermediate host of a parasite, in which the parasite does not undergo any development or replication, but remains, usually encysted, until the paratenic host is ingested by the definitive host of the parasite.

PARITY The status of a woman as regards the fact of having borne viable children. The number of full-term children previously borne by a woman, excluding miscarriages or abortions in early pregnancy, but including stillbirths.

PARTICULARIZATION A method of analysis opposite to generalization or abstraction. It focuses on the specificity of a number of facts and illustrates an issue through the use of example.

PASSAGE The transfer of micro-organisms from human to animal host(s) either directly or via laboratory culture; in the laboratory, this procedure is used to establish the Henle-Koch postulates.

PASSENGER VARIABLE A variable that varies systematically with the dependent variable under study, without being causally related to it; a third (explanatory) variable, the common cause of both the dependent and the passenger variable, "explains" or accounts for their association.

PASSIVE SMOKING See INVOLUNTARY SMOKING

PASTEUR, LOUIS (1822–1895) A French chemist and biologist. One of the founders of bacteriology and therefore an important figure also in epidemiology. Starting in chemistry, he worked out the biological basis for fermentation, and then went on to make many important discoveries in bacteriology, notably vaccines against anthrax and rabies. He is, of course, eponymously honored by the word "pasteurization."

PATH ANALYSIS A mode of analysis involving assumptions about the direction of causal relationships between linked sequences and configurations of variables. This permits the analyst to construct and test the appropriateness of alternative models (in the form of a path diagram) of the causal relations that may exist within the array of variables included in the finite system studied. Identification of the less probable sequences of causal pathways may permit them to be eliminated from further consideration.

PATHOGEN Organism capable of causing disease (literally, causing a pathological process).

PATHOGENESIS The postulated mechanisms by which the etiologic agent produces disease. The difference between ETIOLOGY and pathogenesis should be noted: The etiology of a disease or disability consists of the postulated causes that initiate the pathogenetic mechanisms; control of these causes might lead to prevention of the disease.

PATHOGENICITY The property of an organism that determines the extent to which overt disease is produced in an infected population, or the power of an organism to produce disease. Also used to describe comparable properties of toxic chemicals, etc. Pathogenicity of infectious agents is measured by the ratio of the number of persons developing clinical illness to the number exposed to infection. See also VIR-ULENCE, with which pathogenicity is sometimes confused.

PEARSON, KARL (1857–1936) British mathematician, biologist and geneticist. Pearson was a pupil of Francis Galton, who led the science of statistics further into applications in biology and genetics. He founded the journal *Biometrika,* coined the word "biometry," and taught the next generation of statistician/epidemiologists, including Major Greenwood, Raymond Pearl, and others.

PEARSON'S PRODUCT MOMENT CORRELATION See CORRELATION COEFFICIENT.

PEDIGREE A diagram showing the ancestral relationships and transmission of genetic traits over several generations of a family.

PEER REVIEW Process of review of research proposals, manuscripts submitted for publication, abstracts submitted for presentation at scientific meetings, whereby these are judged for scientific and technical merit by other scientists in the same field. Also refers to review of clinical performance, when it is a form of medical audit.

PENETRANCE The frequency, expressed as a percentage, with which individuals of a given phenotype manifest at least some degree of a specific mutant phenotype associated with a trait. See also GENETIC PENETRANCE.

PERCEIVED NEED A felt need. The term usually refers to need for health care that is felt by the person or community concerned, but which may not be perceived by health professionals.

PERCENTILE The set of divisions that produce exactly 100 equal parts in a series of continuous values, such as children's heights or weights. Thus a child above the 90th percentile has a greater value for height or weight than over 90% of all in the series.

PERINATAL MORTALITY Literally, mortality around the time of birth. Conventionally this time is limited to the period between 28 weeks gestation and one week postnatal. However, as the following discussion indicates, other factors, especially the weight of the fetus, should be considered. The *Ninth (1975) Revision of the International Classification of Diseases* includes the following:

Perinatal mortality statistics

It is recommended that national perinatal statistics should include all fetuses and infants delivered weighing at least 500 g (or, when birth weight is unavailable, the corresponding gestational age [22 weeks] or body length [25 cm crown–heel]), whether alive or dead. It is recognized that legal requirements in many countries may set different criteria for registration purposes, but it is hoped that countries will arrange the registration or reporting procedures in such a way that the events required for inclusion in the statistics can be identified easily. It is further recommended that less mature fetuses and infants should be excluded from perinatal statistics unless there are legal or other valid reasons to the contrary.

It is recommended above that national statistics would include fetuses and infants weighing between 500 g and 1000 g both for their inherent value and because their inclusion improves the completeness of reporting at 1000 g and over.

Inclusion of this group of very immature births, however, disrupts international comparisons because of differences in national practices concerning their registration. Another factor affecting international comparisons is that all live-born infants, irrespective of birth weight, are included in the calculation of rates, whereas some lower limit of maturity is applied to infants born dead.

In order to eliminate these factors, it is recommended that countries should present, solely for international comparisons, "standard perinatal statistics" in which both the numerator and denominator of all rates are restricted to fetuses and infants weighing 1000 g or more (or, where birth weight is unavailable, the corresponding gestational age [28 weeks] or body length [25 cm crown–heel]).

PERINATAL MORTALITY RATE In most industrially developed nations, this is defined as

$$\frac{\text{Perinatal}}{\text{mortality rate}} = \frac{\text{Fetal deaths (28 weeks + of gestation) + postnatal deaths (first week)}}{\text{Fetal deaths (28 weeks + of gestation) + live births}} \times 1000$$

The World Health Organization's definition, more appropriate in nations with less well-established vital records, is

$$\frac{\text{Perinatal}}{\text{mortality rate}} = \frac{\text{Late fetal deaths (28 weeks + of gestation) + postnatal deaths (first week)}}{\text{Live births in a year}} \times 1000$$

Note the differences in denominator of the perinatal mortality rate as defined by WHO and in industrially developed nations. This makes international comparison difficult. The WHO Expert Committee on the Prevention of Perinatal Mortality and Morbidity (1970) recommended a more precise formulation: "Late fetal and early neonatal deaths weighing over 1000 g at birth expressed as a ratio per 1000 live births weighing over 1000 g at birth."

PERIODIC (MEDICAL) EXAMINATIONS Assessment of health status conducted at predetermined intervals, e.g., annually or at specified milestones in life such as infancy, school entry, preemployment, or preretirement. This form of medical examination generally follows a formal protocol, e.g., employing a set of structured questions and/or a predetermined set of laboratory tests.

PERIOD OF COMMUNICABILITY See COMMUNICABLE PERIOD.

PERMISSIBLE EXPOSURE LIMIT (PEL) An occupational health standard to safeguard employees against dangerous chemicals or contaminants in the workplace. See SAFETY STANDARDS.

PERSONAL HEALTH CARE Those services to individuals that are performed on a one-to-one basis by a health care worker for the purpose of maintaining or restoring health.

PERSONAL MONITORING DEVICE An instrument attached to a person to measure the exposure of that person to hazardous substance(s).

PERSON-TIME A measurement combining persons and time, used as denominator in person-time incidence and mortality rates. It is the sum of individual units of time that the persons in the study population have been exposed to the condition of interest. A variant is person-distance, e.g., as in passenger-kilometers. The most frequently used person-time is person-years. With this approach, each subject contributes only as many years of observation to the population at risk as he is actually observed; if he leaves after one year, he contributes one person-year; if after ten, ten person-years. The method can be used to measure incidence over extended and variable time periods.

PERSON-TIME INCIDENCE RATE (Syn: interval incidence density) A measure of the incidence rate of an event, e.g., a disease or death, in a population at risk, given by

$$\frac{\text{Number of events occurring during the interval}}{\text{Number of person-time units at risk observed during the interval}}$$

PERSON-TO-PERSON SPREAD OF DISEASE (Syn: prosodemic) See TRANSMISSION OF INFEC-
TION.

PERSON-YEARS See PERSON-TIME.

PETTY, WILLIAM (1623–1687) A member of the same circle as John Graunt, he is equally
recognized as a pioneer in vital statistics and economics. His ideas and concepts of
lifetime earning capability are contained in *Political Arithmetic* (London, 1691).

PHARMACOEPIDEMIOLOGY The study of the distribution and determinants of drug-related
events in populations, and the application of this study to efficaceous drug treatment.

PHYSICIAN (Syn: medical practitioner, doctor) Professional person qualified by education and authorized by law to practice medicine.

PIE CHART A circular diagram divided into segments, each representing a category or
subset of data. The amount for each category is proportional to the angle sub-
tended at the center of the circle and hence to the area of the sector.

When several pie charts are used to describe several populations, the area of each
circle is proportional to the size of the population it represents.

PILOT INVESTIGATION, STUDY A small-scale test of the methods and procedures to be
used on a larger scale if the pilot study demonstrates that these methods and procedures can work.

PLACEBO, PLACEBO EFFECT An inert medication or procedure. The placebo effect (usually but not necessarily beneficial) is attributable to the expectation that the regimen
will have an effect, i.e., the effect is due to the power of suggestion. See also HALO
EFFECT.

POINT SOURCE EPIDEMIC See EPIDEMIC, COMMON SOURCE.

POISSON DISTRIBUTION A distribution function used to describe the occurrence of rare
events or to describe the sampling distribution of isolated counts in a continuum of
time or space (e.g., sample counts of radioactive disintegration per minute). The
number of events has a Poisson distribution with parameter λ (lambda) if the probability of observing k events ($k = 0, 1, \ldots$) is equal to

$$p(x = k) = \frac{e^{-\lambda}\lambda^k}{k!}$$

where e is the base of natural logarithm, 2.7183. . . . The mean and variance of
the distribution are both equal to λ. This distribution is used in modeling person-
time incidence rates.

POLLUTION Any undesirable modification of air, water, or food by substance(s) that are
toxic or may have adverse effects on health or that are offensive though not necessarily harmful to health.

POLYGENIC INHERITANCE The transmission of a phenotypic trait whose expression depends upon the additive effect of a number of genes.

PONDERAL INDEX The anthropometric index of body mass. Defined as height divided
by the cube root of the body weight. The BODY MASS INDEX is generally regarded as
a better index of body mass.

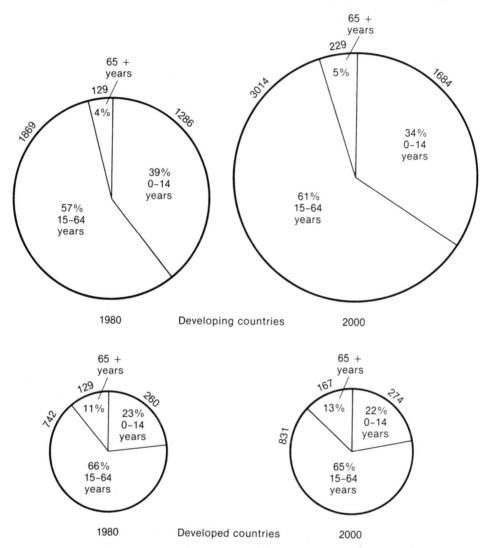

Pie charts of age structure of the population.
(Figures outside the circle show the population in millions.)
From World Health Organization.

POPULATION
1. All the inhabitants of a given country or area considered together; the number of inhabitants of a given country or area.
2. (In sampling) The whole collection of units from which a sample may be drawn; not necessarily a population of persons; the units may be institutions, records, or events. The sample is intended to give results that are representative of the whole population.

POPULATION ATTRIBUTABLE RISK (PAR) This term is used by many epidemiologists[1,2,3] in preference to the terms "attributable fraction (population)" or "etiologic fraction (population)." It is the incidence of a disease in a population that is associated with (attributable to) exposure to the risk factor. It is often expressed as a percentage. It is calculated by similar methods to those described for attributable fraction (population), i.e.,

$$PAR\% = \frac{P_e(I_e - I_u)}{P_t \times I_t} \times 100$$

where P_e = number of persons exposed
P_t = persons in the population
I_e = incidence rate among the exposed
I_u = incidence rate among the unexposed
I_t = incidence rate for the total population

In a case-control study, PAR can be estimated in various ways; Cole and Mac-Mahon[3] give the following formula:

$$PAR\% = \frac{P_e(RR - 1)}{1 + P_e(RR - 1)} \times 100$$

where P_e = proportion of controls exposed
RR = relative risk for exposed, compared to risk of 1 for the unexposed.

[1] MacMahon B, Pugh TF: *Epidemiology; Principles and Methods.* Boston: Little, Brown, 1970.
[2] Fletcher RH, Fletcher SW, Wagner EH: *Clinical Epidemiology—the Essentials.* Baltimore: Williams & Wilkins, 1982.
[3] Cole P, MacMahon B: Attributable risk percent in case-control studies. *Brit J Prev Soc Med* 25:242–244, 1971.

POPULATION ATTRIBUTABLE RISK PERCENT This is the attributable fraction in the population, expressed as a percentage. See also ATTRIBUTABLE FRACTION (POPULATION).

POPULATION BASED Pertaining to a general population defined by geopolitical boundaries; this population is the denominator and/or the sampling frame.

POPULATION DYNAMICS Changes in the structure of a population; loosely used as a synonym for demography.

POPULATION EXCESS RATE A measure of the amount of disease associated with exposure to a putative cause of the disease in the population. It is the difference between the rates of disease in the entire population and among the nonexposed.

POPULATION MEDICINE See COMMUNITY MEDICINE.

POPULATION MOMENTUM In a growing population, the phenomenon of continuing population growth beyond the time when replacement level fertility has been achieved, because of the increasing size of child-bearing and younger age cohorts, resulting from higher fertility and/or falling mortality in preceding years.

POPULATION PYRAMID A graphic presentation of the age and sex composition of the population. The population pyramid is constructed by computing the percentage distribution of a population, simultaneously cross-classified by sex and age. The percentage that each female age group is of the total is plotted on the right and the corresponding percentages for males are plotted on the left. A population pyramid is intended to provide a quick overall comprehension of age and sex structure in the population. A population whose pyramid has a broad base and narrow apex may be identified as a high fertility population. Changing shape over time reflects the changing composition of the population, associated with changes in fertility and mortality at each age.

Since the figure is two dimensional, the word "pyramid" is incorrectly used, but the more accurate word "profile" has never caught on.

Mexico 1970

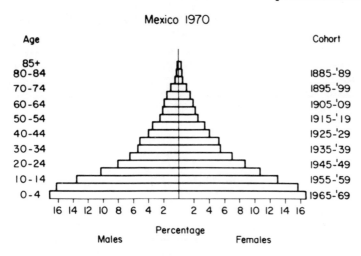

Sweden 1970

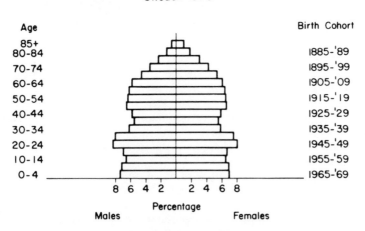

Population pyramids.
Top: High fertility, low proportion survive to old age (Mexico).
Bottom: Low fertility, high proportion survive to old age (Sweden).
From Last, 1980.

POPULATION, STUDY The group selected for investigation.

POPULATION, TARGET The group from which a study population is selected.

POSTERIOR ODDS, POSTERIOR PROBABILITY Probability calculated after reference to results of a study. See BAYES THEOREM.

POSTMARKETING SURVEILLANCE A procedure implemented after a drug has been licenced for public use, designed to provide information on the actual use of the drug for a given indication, and on the occurrence of side effects, adverse reactions, etc. A method for epidemiologic study of adverse drug reactions.

POSTNEONATAL MORTALITY RATE The number of infant deaths between 28 days and one year of age in a given year per 1000 live births in that year. It is an important rate to monitor in developing countries where older infants frequently die of infections and malnutrition.

POTENCY The strength of a particular drug, toxin, or hazard; the ratio of the dose of a standard amount required to elicit a specific response, to the dose of the test agent that elicits the same response.

POTENTIAL YEARS OF LIFE LOST (PYLL) A measure of the relative impact of various diseases and lethal forces on society. PYLL highlights the loss to society as a result of youthful or early deaths. The figure for potential years of life lost due to a particular cause is the sum, over all persons dying from that cause, of the years that these persons would have lived had they experienced normal life expectation. The concept derives from Petty's *Political Arithmetic* (1687) and is elaborated upon in Dublin and Lotka's *Money Value of a Man* (1930).

POWER A characteristic of a statistical hypothesis test, denoting the probability that the null hypothesis will be rejected if it is indeed false. It is equal to 1 minus the probability of type II error. See also ERROR, RESOLUTION. Resolving power is the comparable property of individual measurements.

PRAGMATIC STUDY A study whose aim is to improve health status or health care of a specified population, provide a basis for decisions about health care, or evaluate previous actions. See also EXPLANATORY STUDY; COMMUNITY DIAGNOSIS; PROGRAM REVIEW.

PRECISION

1. The quality of being sharply defined or stated. One measure of precision is the number of distinguishable alternatives from which a measurement was selected, sometimes indicated by the number of significant digits in the measurement. Another measure of precision is the standard error of measurement, the standard deviation of a series of replicate determinations of the same quantity. Precision does not imply accuracy. See also MEASUREMENT, PROBLEMS WITH TERMINOLOGY.

2. In statistics, precision is defined as the inverse of the variance of a measurement or estimate.

PRECURSOR An early stage in the course of a disease, or a condition or state preceding pathological onset of a disease; sometimes detectable by SCREENING; may be identified as a RISK MARKER.

PREDICTIVE VALUE In screening and diagnostic tests, the probability that a person with a positive test is a true positive (i.e., does have the disease) is referred to as the "predictive value of a positive test." The predictive value of a negative test is the probability that a person with a negative test does not have the disease. The predictive value of a screening test is determined by the sensitivity and specificity of the test, and by the prevalence of the condition for which the test is used. See also SCREENING; SENSITIVITY AND SPECIFICITY.

PREMUNITION A term used mainly in the epidemiology of parastic diseases, especially malaria. It signifies a state of resistance, in a host harboring a parasite, to superinfection by a parasite of the same species. This state is dependent on the continued survival of parasites in the body and disappears after their elimination. It may be complete or partial.

PREPATENT PERIOD In parasitology, the period equivalent to the incubation period of microbial infections; the corresponding phase may be biologically different from microbial multiplication when the invading organism is a multicellular parasite that undergoes developmental stages in the host.

PRESCRIPTIVE SCREENING See SCREENING.

PREVALENCE The number of instances of a given disease or other condition in a given population at a designated time; sometimes used to mean PREVALENCE RATE. When used without qualification the term usually refers to the situation at a specified point in time (point prevalence).

    prevalence, annual (An occasionally used index) The total number of persons with the disease or attribute at any time during a year. It includes cases of the disease arising before but extending into or through the year as well as those having their inception during the year.

    prevalence, lifetime The total number of persons known to have had the disease or attribute for at least part of their life.

    prevalence, period The total number of persons known to have had the disease or attribute at any time during a specified period.

    prevalence, point The number of persons with a disease or an attribute at a specified point in time.

PREVALENCE RATE (RATIO) The total number of all individuals who have an attribute or disease at a particular time (or during a particular period) divided by the population at risk of having the attribute or disease at this point in time or midway through the period. A problem may arise with calculating period prevalence rates because of the difficulty of defining the most appropriate denominator. See also PREVALENCE.

PREVALENCE STUDY See CROSS-SECTIONAL STUDY.

PREVENTABLE FRACTION (population) In a situation in which exposure to a given factor is believed to protect against a disease (or other outcome), the preventable fraction in the population is the proportion of the disease (in the population) that would be prevented if the whole population were exposed to the factor. This value must be interpreted with caution, as part or all of the apparent protective effect may be due to other factors associated with the apparent protective factor.

    In a study of a total population, the preventable fraction (population) is computed as $\dfrac{I_p - I_e}{I_p}$, where I_p is the incidence rate of the disease (or other outcome) in the population, and I_e is the incidence rate in the exposed persons in the population.

PREVENTED FRACTION (population) In a situation in which exposure to a given factor is believed to protect against a disease (or other outcome), the prevented fraction is the proportion of the hypothetical total load of disease (in the population) that has been prevented by exposure to the factor. This value must be interpreted with caution, as part or all of the apparent protective effect may be due to other factors associated with the apparent protective factor.

    In a study of a total population the prevented fraction is computed as $\dfrac{I_u - I_p}{I_u}$, where I_p is the rate of the disease in the population, and I_u is the rate among people unexposed to the factor.

PREVENTION The goals of medicine are to promote health, to preserve health, to restore health when it is impaired, and to minimize suffering and distress. These goals are embodied in the word "prevention," which is easiest to define in the context of levels, customarily called primary, secondary, and tertiary prevention. Authorities on PREVENTIVE MEDICINE do not agree on the precise boundaries between these levels, nor on how many levels can be distinguished, but the differences of opinion are semantic rather than substantive.

    An epidemiologic interpretation of the distinction between primary and secondary prevention is that primary prevention is aimed at reducing incidence of disease and other departures from good health, secondary prevention aims to reduce prevalence by shortening the duration, and tertiary prevention is aimed at reducing complications.

Primary prevention can be defined as the protection of health by personal and community-wide effects, e.g., preserving good nutritional status, physical fitness, and emotional well-being, immunizing against infectious diseases, and making the environment safe. (But see also HEALTH PROMOTION.)

Secondary prevention can be defined as the measures available to individuals and populations for the early detection and prompt and effective intervention to correct departures from good health.

Tertiary prevention consists of the measures available to reduce or eliminate long-term impairments and disabilities, minimize suffering caused by existing departures from good health, and to promote the patient's adjustment to irremediable conditions. This extends the concept of prevention into the field of rehabilitation.

PREVENTIVE MEDICINE The application of preventive measures by clinical practitioners. A specialized field of medical practice composed of distinct disciplines that utilize skills focusing on the health of defined populations in order to promote and maintain health and well-being and prevent disease, disability, and premature death.

In addition to the knowledge of basic and clinical sciences and the skills common to all physicians, the distinctive aspects of preventive medicine include knowledge of and competence in biostatistics, epidemiology, administration including planning, organization, management, financing, and evaluation of health programs; environmental health; application of social and behavioral factors in health and disease; and the application of primary, secondary, and tertiary prevention measures within clinical medicine. (The above is the definition and description of the field that has been adopted by the American College of Preventive Medicine; for completeness, at least two other items ought to be added, i.e., health education and nutrition).

PRIMARY CASE The individual who introduces the disease into the family or group under study. Not necessarily the first diagnosed case in a family or group. See also INDEX CASE.

PRIMARY HEALTH CARE
1. Health care that begins at the time of first encounter between a patient and a provider of health care; An alternative term is primary medical care.
2. The WHO definition of primary health care includes much more: Primary health care is essential health care made accessible at a cost the country and the community can afford, with methods that are practical, scientifically sound, and socially acceptable. Everyone in the community should have access to it, and everyone should be involved in it. Related sectors should also be involved in it in addition to the health sector. At the very least it should include education of the community on the health problems prevalent and on methods of preventing health problems from arising or of controlling them; the promotion of adequate supplies of food and of proper nutrition; sufficient safe water and basic sanitation; maternal and child health care including family planning; the prevention and control of locally endemic diseases; immunization against the main infectious diseases; appropriate treatment of common diseases and injuries; and the provision of essential drugs. (From *Glossary of Terms Used in the Health for All Series No. 1–8.* Geneva: WHO, 1984.)

PRINCIPAL COMPONENT ANALYSIS A statistical method to simplify the description of a set of interrelated variables. Its general objectives are data reduction and interpretation; there is no separation into dependent and independent variables; the original set of correlated variables is transformed into a smaller set of uncorrelated variables called the principal components. Often used as the first step in a factor analysis.

PRIOR PROBABILITY Probability calculated or estimated from theory or belief, before a study is done. See BAYES' THEOREM.

PROBABILITY

1. The limit of the relative frequency of an event in a sequence of N random trials as N approaches infinity, i.e., the limit of

$$\frac{\text{Number of occurrence of the event}}{N}$$

2. A measure, ranging from zero to 1, of the degree of belief in a hypothesis or statement.

PROBABILITY DENSITY The frequency distribution of a continuous random variable.

PROBABILITY DISTRIBUTION For a discrete random variable, the function that gives the probabilities that the variable equals each of a sequence of possible values. Examples include the binomial and Poisson distributions. For a continuous random variable, often used synonymously with the probability density function.

PROBABILITY SAMPLE (Syn: random sample) See SAMPLE.

PROBABILITY THEORY The branch of mathematics dealing with the purely logical properties of probability. Its theorems underly most statistical methods.

PROBAND See PROPOSITUS.

PROBLEM-ORIENTED MEDICAL RECORD (POMR) A medical record in which the patient's history, physical findings, laboratory results, etc., are organized to give a cumulative record of problems, e.g., hemoptysis, rather than disease, e.g., pneumonia. The record includes subjective, objective, and significant negative information, discussions and conclusions, and diagnostic and treatment plans with respect to each problem. The record, which was developed by Lawrence Weed,[1] contrasts with the traditional medical record, which is less formally organized, usually recording all information from each source (history, physical, and laboratory findings) together without regard to the problems the information describes.

Since the problems may not be described in terms of conventional disease labels, their classification and counting for epidemiologic purposes are sometimes difficult. The INTERNATIONAL CLASSIFICATION OF HEALTH PROBLEMS IN PRIMARY CARE (ICHPPC) is an attempt to overcome this difficulty.

[1] Weed LL: Medical records that guide and teach. *New Engl J Med* 278:593–600, 652–657, 1968.

PROCATARCTIC CAUSE A term used by epidemiologists of the late 19th and early 20th centuries, probably last used by GREENWOOD, to describe predisposing causes associated with habits of life.

PROFESSIONAL ACTIVITY STUDY (PAS) The HOSPITAL DISCHARGE ABSTRACT SYSTEM that covers many acute short-stay hospitals in the United States. It provides regularly published statistical tables arranged according to hospital service, diagnostic category, etc., giving details on diagnostic and therapeutic procedures, length of stay and outcome.

PROGRAM

1. A (formal) set of procedures to conduct an activity, e.g., control of malaria.
2. An ordered list of instructions directing a computer to carry out a desired sequence of operations. The objective is normally the solution of a problem.

PROGRAM EVALUATION AND REVIEW TECHNIQUES (PERT) A work-scheduling method that uses ALGORITHMS and also enunciates general principles of procedure for allocating resources. Calls for listing specific tasks to be completed and the resources—personnel, equipment, supplies, and other items—that will be needed, along with their costs, a time chart indicating when each component task is to begin and end, giving interim accomplishment levels during that period, and a specification of times for interim review of the progress of the plan.

PROGRAM REVIEW An evaluative study of a specific health program operating in a specific setting, performed to provide a basis for decisions concerning the operation of the program.

PROGRAM TRIAL An experimental or quasi-experimental evaluative study of a (health) program.

PROLECTIVE Pertaining to data collected by planning in advance. Contrast retrolective. The terms prolective and retrolective, coined by AR Feinstein[1] are said to describe more precisely the actions of research workers than the common terms prospective and retrospective; use of these terms is limited, and is deprecated by many epidemiologists.

[1] *Clin Pharmacol Ther* 30:564–577, 1981.

PROPORTION A type of ratio in which the numerator is included in the denominator. The ratio of a part to the whole, expressed as a "decimal fraction" (e.g., 0.2), as a "vulgar fraction" ($\frac{1}{5}$), or, loosely, as a percentage (20%). By definition, a proportion (p) must be in the range (decimal) $0.0 \leq p \leq 1.0$. Since numerator and denominator have the same dimension, any dimensional contents cancel out, and a proportion is a dimensionless quantity. Where numerator and denominator are based upon counts rather than upon measurements, the originals are also dimensionless, although it should be understood that proportions can be used for measured quantities, e.g., the skin area of the lower limb is x percent of the total skin area, as well as for counts, e.g., 0.15 of the population died. A prevalence rate is a count-based proportion. The nondimensionality of a proportion, and its range limitations, do not necessarily apply to other kinds of ratios, of which "proportion" is a subset. See also RATE; RATIO.

PROPORTIONAL HAZARDS MODEL (Syn: Cox model) A statistical MODEL in SURVIVAL ANALYSIS that asserts that the effect of the study factors on the HAZARD RATE in the study population is multiplicative and does not change over time. For example, the model for two factors x_1 and x_2 asserts that the rate at time t λ (t), is given by

$$e^{\beta_1 x_1 + \beta_2 x_3} \lambda_0(t)$$

where $\lambda_0(t)$ is the rate when $x_1 = x_2 = 0$, and e is the (natural) exponential function.

PROPORTIONATE MORTALITY RATE, RATIO (PMR) Number of deaths from a given cause in a specified time period, per 100 or 1000 total deaths in the same time period. Can give rise to misleading conclusions if used to compare mortality experience of populations with different distributions of causes of death.

PROPOSITUS (Syn: proband) The family member who first draws attention to a (genetic) pedigree of a given trait. The INDEX CASE in a genetic study.

PROSPECTIVE STUDY See COHORT STUDY.

PROTOCOL The plan, or set of steps, to be followed in a study or investigation, or in an intervention program. See also ALGORITHM, CLINICAL.

PROXIMATE DETERMINANT OF FERTILITY Factor having a direct influence on fertility; such factors include age at marriage, breastfeeding, abortion, and contraceptive use.

PUBLIC HEALTH Public health is one of the efforts organized by society to protect, promote, and restore the people's health. It is the combination of sciences, skills, and beliefs that is directed to the maintenance and improvement of the health of all the people through collective or social actions. The programs, services, and institutions involved emphasize the prevention of disease and the health needs of the population as a whole. Public health activities change with changing technology and social values, but the goals remain the same: to reduce the amount of disease, premature death, and disease-produced discomfort and disability in the population. Public health is thus a social institution, a discipline, and a practice.

PUNCH CARD A card on which data are stored by means of holes punched in specified positions; useful in storing, processing, and analyzing data. Edge-punch cards have marginal holes converted to slots by punching so that they can be manually sorted. The commonly used variety of punch cards have 80 columns and 12 rows. In each column of the card there are 12 positions at which holes may be punched, according to a predetermined code. The position of the hole is the means of identifying the value of a variable. Punch cards of this type are sorted mechanically or electrically to provide a rapid means of processing and analyzing data, sometimes of great complexity. See also DATA PROCESSING.

P VALUE See P (PROBABILITY).

Q

QALY Acronym for quality-adjusted life years; this is an adjustment of life expectancy that allows for prevalence of activity-limitation, assessed from hospital discharge data or by health survey data, in the population subgroup for which QALY is calculated. For example, the life expectancy of males at birth in Canada in 1978 was 70.8 years; after adjusting for activity-limitation using health survey data, quality-adjusted life expectancy, or QALY, was 65.8 years.[1]

[1] Wilkins R, Adams O: *Healthfulness of Life.* Montreal, 1983.

QUALITATIVE DATA Observations or information characterized by measurement on a categorical scale, i.e., a dichotomous or nominal scale, or, if the categories are ordered, an ordinal scale. Examples are sex, hair color, death or survival, and nationality. See also MEASUREMENT SCALE.

QUALITY CONTROL The supervision and control of all operations involved in a process, usually involving sampling and inspection, in order to detect and correct systematic or excessively random variations in quality.

QUALITY OF CARE A level of performance or accomplishment that characterizes the health care provided. Ultimately, measures of the quality of care always depend upon value judgments, but there are ingredients and determinants of quality that can be measured objectively. These ingredients and determinants have been classified by Donabedian[1] into measures of structure (e.g., manpower, facilities), process (e.g., diagnostic and therapeutic procedures), and outcome (e.g., case fatality rates, disability rates, and levels of patient satisfaction with the service). See also HEALTH SERVICES RESEARCH.

[1] Donabedian A: *A Guide to Medical Care Administration* (Vol. 2). New York: American Public Health Association, 1969.

QUALITY OF LIFE In a general sense, that which makes life worth living. In a more "quantitative" sense, an estimate of remaining life free of impairment, disability or handicap, as used in the expression "quality adjusted life years;" somewhere between these is an estimate of the utility of life—for instance, in clinical decision analysis, the utility of life that is impaired by a disabling degree of angina pectoris may be compared with that of a life that may be shorter in duration but free of disabling pain, as a result of applying therapeutic procedures. Such trade-offs are part of clinical decision analysis. See also UTILITY.

QUANTILES Divisions of a distribution into equal, ordered subgroups. Deciles are tenths; quartiles, quarters; quintiles, fifths; terciles, thirds; and centiles, hundredths.

QUANTITATIVE DATA Data in numerical quantities such as continuous measurements or counts.

QUARANTINE The 14th edition of *Control of Communicable Disease in Man*[1] gives the following:

Restriction of the activities of well persons or animals who have been exposed to a case of communicable disease during its period of communicability (i.e., contacts) to prevent disease transmission during the incubation period if infection should occur.

   a) Absolute or complete quarantine: The limitation of freedom of movement of those exposed to a communicable disease for a period of time not longer than the longest usual incubation period of that disease, in such manner as to prevent effective contact with those not so exposed (see Isolation).

   b) Modified quarantine: A selective, partial limitation of freedom of movement of contacts, commonly on the basis of known or presumed differences in susceptibility and related to the danger of disease transmission. It may be designed to meet particular situations. Examples are exclusion of children from school, exemption of immune persons from provisions applicable to susceptible persons, or restriction of military populations to the post or to quarters. It includes: Personal surveillance, the practice of close medical or other supervision of contacts in order to permit prompt recognition of infection or illness but without restricting their movements; and Segregation, the separation of some part of a group of persons or domestic animals from the others for special consideration, control or observation—removal of susceptible children to homes of immune persons, or establishment of a sanitary boundary to protect uninfected from infected portions of a population.

   See also ISOLATION.

[1] Washington DC: American Public Health Association, 1985.

QUASI-EXPERIMENT An experiment in which the investigator lacks full control over the allocation and/or the timing of the intervention.

QUESTIONNAIRE A predetermined set of questions used to collect data—clinical data, social status, occupational group, etc. This term is often applied to a self-completed survey instrument, as contrasted with an INTERVIEW SCHEDULE.

QUETELET, LAMBERT ADOLPHE JACQUES (1796–1857) Belgian astronomer, statistician, and social scientist, one of the first to apply statistical thinking to the social and biological sciences, e.g., in delineating the (normal) distribution of variables such as height in the population. He influenced others who followed, e.g., FLORENCE NIGHTINGALE.

QUETELET'S INDEX See BODY MASS INDEX.

QUOTA SAMPLING A method by which the proportions in the sample in various subgroups (according to criteria such as age, sex, and social status of the individuals to be selected) are chosen to agree with the corresponding proportions in the population. The resulting sample may not be representative of characteristics that have not been taken into account.

QUOTIENT The result of the division of a numerator by a denominator.

R

RACE Persons who are relatively homogeneous with respect to biological inheritance. See also ETHNIC GROUP.

RADIX The hypothetical size of the birth cohort in a life table, commonly 1000 or 100,000.

RAHE–HOLMES SOCIAL READJUSTMENT RATING SCALE See LIFE EVENTS.

RAMAZZINI, BERNARDINO (1633–1714) An Italian physician, "Father of Occupational Medicine;" he published *De Morbis Artificum* (On the Diseases of Workers) in 1700. Based on observation and anecdote, this was the first systematic account of diseases related to workplace exposures.

RANDOM Governed by chance; not completely determined by other factors. As opposed to deterministic.

RANDOM ALLOCATION See RANDOMIZATION.

RANDOMIZATION Allocation of individuals to groups, e.g., for experimental and control regimens, by chance. Within the limits of chance variation, randomization should make the control and experimental groups similar at the start of an investigation and ensure that personal judgment and prejudices of the investigator do not influence allocation.

Randomization or random assignment should not be confused with haphazard assignment. Random assignment follows a predetermined plan that is usually devised with the aid of a table of random numbers. The pattern of assignment may appear to be haphazard, but this arises from the haphazard nature with which digits occur in a table of random numbers, and not from the haphazard whim of the investigator in allocating patients.

RANDOMIZED CONTROLLED TRIAL (RCT) An epidemiologic experiment in which subjects in a population are randomly allocated into groups, usually called "study" and "control" groups, to receive or not to receive an experimental preventive or therapeutic procedure, maneuver, or intervention. The results are assessed by rigorous comparison of rates of disease, death, recovery, or other appropriate outcome in the study and control groups, respectively. Randomized controlled trials are generally regarded as the most scientifically rigorous method of hypothesis testing available in epidemiology. A few authors refer to this method as "randomized control trial." See also EXPERIMENTAL EPIDEMIOLOGY.

RANDOM SAMPLE A sample that is arrived at by selecting sample units such that each possible unit has a fixed and determinate probability of selection. See also SAMPLE.

RANGE OF DISTRIBUTION The difference between the largest and smallest values in a distribution.

RANKING SCALE (Ordinal Scale) A scale that arrays the members of a group from high to low according to the magnitude of the observations, assigns numbers to the ranks, and neglects distances between members of the array.

RATE A rate is a measure of the frequency of a phenomenon. In epidemiology, demography, and vital statistics, a rate is an expression of the frequency with which an event occurs in a defined population; the use of rates rather than raw numbers is essential for comparison of experience between populations at different times, different places, or among different classes of persons.

The components of a rate are the numerator, the denominator, the specified time in which events occur, and usually a multiplier, a power of 10, which converts the rate from an awkward fraction or decimal to a whole number:

$$\text{Rate} = \frac{\text{Number of events in specified period}}{\text{Average population during the period}} \times 10^n$$

All rates are ratios, calculated by dividing a numerator, e.g., the number of deaths, or newly occurring cases of a disease in a given period, by a denominator, e.g., the average population during that period. Some rates are proportions, i.e., the numerator is contained within the denominator. Rate has several different usages in epidemiology.

1. As a synonym for ratio, it refers to proportions as rates, as in the terms cumulative incidence rate, prevalence rate, survival rate (cf. *Webster's Dictionary*, which gives proportion and ratio as synonyms for rate).
2. In other situations, rate refers only to ratios representing relative changes (actual or potential) in two quantities. This accords with the *OED*, which gives "relative amount of variation" among its entries for rate.
3. Sometimes rate is further restricted to refer only to ratios representing changes over time. In this usage, prevalence rate would not be a "true" rate because it cannot be expressed in relation to units of time but only to a "point" in time; in contrast, the force of mortality or force of morbidity (hazard rate) is a "true" rate for it can be expressed as the number of cases developing per unit time, divided by the total size of the population at risk.

RATE DIFFERENCE (RD) The absolute difference between two rates, for example, the difference in incidence rate between a population group exposed to a causal factor and a population group not exposed to the factor:

$$RD = I_e - I_u$$

where I_e = incidence rate among exposed, and I_u = incidence rate among unexposed. In comparisons of exposed and unexposed groups, the term excess rate may be used as a synonym for rate difference.

RATE-ODDS RATIO See ODDS RATIO.

RATE RATIO (RR) The ratio of two rates. The term is used in epidemiologic research with a precise meaning, i.e., the ratio of the rate in the exposed population to the rate in the unexposed population:

$$RR = \frac{I_e}{I_u}$$

where I_e is the incidence rate among exposed, and I_u is the incidence rate among unexposed. See also RELATIVE RISK.

RATIO The value obtained by dividing one quantity by another: a general term of which rate, proportion, percentage, etc., are subsets. The important difference between a proportion and a ratio is that the numerator of a proportion is included in the population defined by the denominator, whereas this is not necessarily so for a ratio. A ratio is an expression of the relationship between a numerator and a denominator where the two usually are separate and distinct quantities, neither being included in the other.

The dimensionality of a ratio is obtained through algebraic cancellation, summation, etc., of the dimensionalities of its numerator and denominator terms. Both counted and measured values may be included in the numerator and in the denominator. There are no general restrictions on the dimensionalities or ranges of ratios, as there are in some of its subsets (e.g., proportion, prevalence). Ratios are sometimes expressed as percentages (e.g., standardized mortality ratio, FEV_1 percent). In these cases, unlike the special case of a PROPORTION, the value may exceed 100. See also PROPORTION; RATE.

RATIO SCALE See MEASUREMENT SCALE.

RECEIVER OPERATING CHARACTERISTIC (ROC) CURVE (Syn: relative operating characteristic curve) A graphic means for assessing the ability of a screening test to discriminate between healthy and diseased persons. The term "receiver operating characteristic" comes from psychometry where the characteristic operating response of a receiver-individual to faint stimuli or nonstimuli was recorded.

RECORD LINKAGE A method for assembling the information contained in two or more records, e.g., in different sets of medical charts, and in vital records such as birth and death certificates, and a procedure to ensure that the same individual is counted only once. This procedure incorporates a unique identifying system such as a personal identification number and/or birth name(s) of the individual's mother.

Record linkage makes it possible to relate significant health events that are remote from one another in time and place or to bring together records of different individuals, e.g., members of a family. The resulting information is generally stored and retrieved by computer, which can be programmed to tabulate and analyze the data.

"Each person in the world creates a book of life. This book starts with birth and ends with death. Its pages are made of the records of the principal events in life. Record linkage is the name given to the process of assembling the pages of this book into a volume."[1]

[1] Dunn HL: Record linkage. *Am J Pub Health* 36:1412, 1946

RECRUDESCENCE Reactivation of infection.

REED, WALTER (1851–1902) US Army physician and epidemiologist. Responsible for epidemiologic investigations and experiments that established the transmission of yellow fever by a filterable virus carried by culicine mosquitoes. The rigorous logic applied to both the experimental and incidental observations by Reed and his colleagues is recognized as one of the great achievements of medical science.

REFERENCE POPULATION The standard against which a population that is being studied can be compared.

REFINEMENT The process of identifying new subcategories of study variables for the purpose of more accurate or more detailed description of relationships. An example is refinement of the concept of serum cholesterol level into high, low, and very low density lipoproteins.

REGISTER, REGISTRY In epidemiology the term "register" is applied to the file of data concerning all cases of a particular disease or other health-relevant condition in a defined population such that the cases can be related to a population base. With this information incidence rates can be calculated. If the cases are regularly followed up, information on remission, exacerbation, prevalence, and survival can also be obtained. The *register* is the actual document, and the *registry* is the system of ongoing registration.

In most developed countries all births and deaths are recorded through birth and death registration systems. Results and summaries are then tabulated and published. Examples of registries that have epidemiologic value include the following:

Cancer registries, which secure reports of cancer patients as soon as possible after first diagnosis. The principal sources for these reports are the hospitals serving the community, but a few cases are not reported until death.

Twin registries, which have provided the basis for studies attempting to differentiate genetic from environmental factors in the etiology of cancer, and other conditions where both genetic and environmental factors may be contributing causes.

Birth defect registries, which seek to document anomalies that are apparent at or soon after birth. They suffer from incompleteness due to omission of stillbirths and of anomalies that do not declare their presence until later in life, such as certain forms of congenital heart lesion, mental deficiency, and neurological disorders.

Other types of registers include blindness and other forms of physical handicap, high-risk infants, persons addicted to drugs, etc. Most of these, however, are not truly population based, but merely list those persons known to or attending some agency or service that provides for them.

REGISTRATION The term "registration" implies something more than notification for the purpose of immediate action or to permit the counting of cases. A register requires that a permanent record be established, including identifying data. Cases may be followed up, and statistical tabulations may be prepared both on frequency and on survival. In addition, the persons listed on a register may be subjects of special studies.

REGRESSION
1. As used by FRANCIS GALTON, regression meant the tendency for offspring of exceptional parents (very tall, very intelligent, etc.) to possess characteristics closer to the average for the general population. (Hence, "regression to the mean.")
2. In statistics, regression is a synonym for REGRESSION ANALYSIS.

REGRESSION ANALYSIS Given data on a dependent variable y and one or more independent variables x_1, x_2, etc. regression analysis involves finding the "best" mathematical model (within some restricted class of models) to describe y as a function of the x's, or to predict y from the x's. The most common form is a linear model; in epidemiology, the logistic and proportional hazards models are also common.

REGRESSION LINE Diagrammatic presentation of a regression equation, usually drawn with the independent variable, x, as the abscissa and the dependent variable, y, as ordinate. Three variables can be shown diagrammatically on an isometric chart or stereogram.

RELATIONSHIP See ASSOCIATION.

RELATIVE ODDS See ODDS RATIO.

RELATIVE RISK
1. The ratio of the RISK of disease or death among the exposed to the risk among the unexposed; this usage is synonymous with RISK RATIO.
2. Alternatively, the ratio of the cumulative incidence rate in the exposed to the cumulative incidence rate in the unexposed, i.e., the cumulative incidence ratio.
3. The term "relative risk" has also been used synonymously with "odds ratio" and, in some biostatistical articles, has been used for the ratio of FORCES OF MORBIDITY. The use of the term "relative risk" for several different quantities arises from the fact that for "rare" diseases (e.g., most cancers) all the quantities approximate one another. For common occurrences (e.g., neonatal mor-

tality in infants under 1500-g birth weight), the approximations do not hold. See also CUMULATIVE INCIDENCE RATIO; ODDS RATIO; RATE RATIO; RISK RATIO.

RELIABILITY The degree of stability exhibited when a measurement is repeated under identical conditions. *Reliability* refers to the degree to which the results obtained by a measurement procedure can be replicated. Lack of reliability may arise from divergences between observers or instruments of measurement or instability of the attribute being measured. See also MEASUREMENT, PROBLEMS WITH TERMINOLOGY; OBSERVER VARIATION.

REPEATABILITY (Syn: reproducibility) A test or measurement is repeatable if the results are identical or closely similar each time it is conducted. See also MEASUREMENT, PROBLEMS WITH TERMINOLOGY; RELIABILITY.

REPLACEMENT LEVEL FERTILITY The level of fertility at which a cohort of women are having only enough daughters to replace themselves in the population. By definition, replacement level fertility is equal to a net reproduction rate of 1.00. The total fertility rate is also used as a measure of replacement level fertility; in the United States today, a total fertility rate of 2.12 is considered to be replacement level; it is higher than 2 because of mortality and because of a sex ratio greater than 1 at birth. The higher the mortality rate, the higher is replacement level fertility.

REPLICATION The execution of an experiment or survey more than once so as to confirm the findings, increase precision, and obtain a closer estimation of sampling error. *Exact replication* should be distinguished from *consistency of results on replication.* Exact replication is often possible in the physical sciences, but in the biological and behavioral sciences, to which epidemiology belongs, consistency of results on replication is often the best that can be attained. Consistency of results on replication is perhaps the most important criterion in judgments of causality.

REPRESENTATIVE SAMPLE The term "representative" as it is commonly used is undefined in the statistical or mathematical sense; it means simply that the sample resembles the population in some way.

The use of probability sampling will not ensure that any single sample will be "representative" of the population in all possible respects. If, for example, it is found that the sample age distribution is quite different from that of the population, it is possible to make corrections for the known differences. A common fallacy lies in the unwarranted assumption that, if the sample resembles the population closely on those factors that have been checked, it is "totally representative" and that no difference exists between the sample and the universe or reference population.

Kendall and Buckland[1] comment as follows: "In the widest sense, a sample which is representative of a population. Some confusion arises according to whether 'representative' is regarded as meaning 'selected by some process which gives all samples an equal chance of appearing to represent the population'; or, alternatively, whether it means 'typical in respect of certain characteristics, however chosen'. On the whole, it seems best to confine the word 'representative' to samples which turn out to be so, however chosen, rather than apply it to those chosen with the object of being representative."

[1] Kendall MG, Buckland WR: *A Dictionary of Statistical Terms,* 4th ed. London: Longman, 1982.

REPRODUCIBILITY See REPEATABILITY.

REPRODUCTIVE ISOLATION Absence of interbreeding between populations.

RESEARCH DESIGN The procedures and methods, predetermined by an investigator, to be adhered to in conducting a research project.

RESERVOIR OF INFECTION

1. Any person, animal, arthropod, plant, soil, or substance, or a combination of

these, in which an infectious agent normally lives and multiplies, on which it depends primarily for survival, and where it reproduces itself in such a manner that it can be transmitted to a susceptible host.

2. The natural habitat of the infectious agent.

RESOLUTION (Syn: resolving power) A component of a measuring instrument that helps determine precision. The degree of refinement of the measuring process is commonly referred to as the "resolution' or the "resolving power of the system." See also POWER. The capability of distinguishing between things that are indeed separate or distinct from one another.

RESOLVING POWER The capacity of a system to distinguish between truly distinct things that are close together.

RESPONSE RATE The number of completed or returned survey instruments (questionnaires, interviews, etc.) divided by the total number of persons who would have been surveyed if all had participated. Usually expressed as a percentage. Nonresponse can have several causes, e.g., death, removal out of the survey community, and refusal. See also BIAS; COMPLETION RATE; NONPARTICIPANTS.

RETROLECTIVE Pertaining to data gathered from medical records or other sources, when data collection took place without prior planning for the needs of an investigation. See also PROLECTIVE; term in limited use.

RETROSPECTIVE STUDY A research design that is used to test etiologic hypotheses in which inferences about exposure to the putative causal factor(s) are derived from data relating to characteristics of the persons under study or to events or experiences in their past. The essential feature is that some of the persons under study have the disease or other outcome condition of interest, and their characteristics and past experiences are compared with those of other, unaffected persons. Persons who differ in the severity of the disease may also be compared. There is disagreement among epidemiologists as to the desirability of using the term "retrospective study" rather than "case control study" to describe this method. See also CASE CONTROL STUDY.

RETROVIRUS This name is given to a family of RNA viruses characterized by the presence of an enzyme, reverse transcriptase, that enables transcription of RNA to DNA inside an affected cell. Thus, retroviruses can make copies of themselves in host cells. The most important retrovirus is the human immunodeficiency virus (HIV); this makes copies of itself in host cells such as T4 "helper" lymphocytes and normal immune responses are disrupted.

RISK The probability that an event will occur, e.g., that an individual will become ill or die within a stated period of time or age. Also, a nontechnical term encompassing a variety of measures of the probability of a (generally) unfavorable outcome. See also PROBABILITY.

RISK ASSESSMENT The qualitative or quantitative estimation of the likelihood of adverse effects that may result from exposure to specified health hazards or from the absence of beneficial influences.

RISK BENEFIT ANALYSIS The process of analyzing and comparing on a single scale the expected positive (benefits) and negative (risks, costs) results of an action, or lack of an action.

RISK BENEFIT RATIO The results of a risk benefit analysis, expressed as the ratio of risks to benefits.

RISK DIFFERENCE (Syn: excess risk) The absolute difference between two risks.

RISK FACTOR An aspect of personal behavior or lifestyle, an environmental exposure, or an inborn or inherited characteristic, which on the basis of epidemiologic evidence is known to be associated with health-related condition(s) considered important to prevent. The term "risk factor" is rather loosely used, with any of the following meanings:

1. An attribute or exposure that is associated with an increased probability of a specified outcome, such as the occurrence of a disease. Not necessarily a causal factor. A RISK MARKER.

2. An attribute or exposure that increases the probability of occurrence of disease or other specified outcome. A DETERMINANT.

3. A determinant that can be modified by intervention, thereby reducing the probability of occurrence of disease or other specified outcomes. To avoid confusion, it may be referred to as a modifiable risk factor.

RISK MANAGEMENT The steps taken to alter, i.e., reduce, the levels of risk to which an individual or a population is subject.

RISK MARKER (Syn: risk indicator) An attribute that is associated with an increased probability of occurrence of a disease or other specified outcome and that can be used as an indicator of this increased risk. Not necessarily a causal factor. See also RISK FACTOR.

RISK RATIO The ratio of two risks.

ROBUST A statistical test or procedure is said to be robust if it is not very sensitive to departures from the assumptions on which it is strictly predicted (e.g., that the data are normally distributed).

ROSS, RONALD (1857–1932) Continued in India the work begun by Laveran and Manson on mosquitoes as vectors of infectious disease. In a series of experiments and microscopic dissections, he concluded that only the anopheles mosquitoes carried the malaria parasite and that a developmental stage of the parasite took place in the mosquito (On some peculiar pigmented cells found in two mosquitoes fed on malarial blood *Brit Med J* 1786–1787, 1897). Awarded the Nobel prize for medicine in 1902.

RUBRIC Section or chapter heading. Used in epidemiology with reference to groups of diseases, e.g., as in the INTERNATIONAL CLASSIFICATION OF DISEASE (ICD).

S

SAFETY FACTOR A multiplicative factor incorporated in risk assessments or safety standards to allow for unpredictable types of variation, such as variability from test animals to humans, random variation within an experiment, and person-to-person variability. Safety factors are often in the range of 10 to 1000.

SAFETY STANDARDS Under the requirements of the Occupational Safety and Health Act (OSHA, 1970), "occupational safety and health standard" means a standard that requires conditions, or the adoption of one or more practices, means, methods, operations, or processes reasonably necessary or appropriate to provide safe or healthful employment and places of employment. Safety standards may be adopted by national consensus or established by federal regulation. These standards have been adopted in many other nations besides the United States, although some European and other countries have their own standards, which may be lower or higher than those in the United States.

There are several varieties of safety standards:
1. OSHA-promulgated, mainly for carcinogens, also for cotton dust and lead. These are Permissable Exposure Limits (PELs).
2. National Institute of Occupational Safety and Health (NIOSH) recommendations, often lower limits, based on animal toxicity tests, empirical observations, epidemiologic investigations; these are Recommended Exposure Limits (RELs).
3. An older-established set of criteria has been set by the American Conference of Governmental Industrial Hygienists; these are Threshhold Limit Values (TLVs) that have now replaced an earlier set of Maximum Allowable Concentrations (MACs).

SAMPLE A selected subset of a population. A sample may be random or nonrandom and may be representative or nonrepresentative. Several types of sample can be distinguished, including the following:

Cluster sample: Each unit selected is a group of persons (all persons in a city block, a family, etc.) rather than an individual.

Grab sample (Syn: sample of convenience): These ill-defined terms describe samples selected by easily employed but basically nonprobabilistic methods. "Man-in-the-street" surveys and a survey of blood pressure among volunteers who drop in at an examination booth in a public place are in this category. It is improper to generalize from the results of a survey based upon such a sample for there is no way of knowing what sorts of bias may have been operating. See also BIAS.

Probability (random) sample: All individuals have a known chance of selection. They may all have an equal chance of being selected, or, if a stratified sampling method is used, the rate at which individuals from several subsets are sampled can be varied so as to produce greater representation of some classes than of others.

A probability sample is created by assigning an identity (label, number) to all individuals in the "universe" population, e.g., by arranging them in alphabetical order and numbering in sequence, or simply assigning a number to each, or by grouping according to area of residence and numbering the groups. The next step

117

is to select individuals (or groups) for study by a procedure such as use of a table of random numbers (or comparable procedure) to ensure that the chance of selection is known.

Simple random sample: In this elementary kind of sample each person has an equal chance of being selected out of the entire population. One way of carrying out this procedure is to assign each person a number, starting with 1, 2, 3, and so on. Then numbers are selected at random, preferably from a table of random numbers, until the desired sample size is attained.

Stratified random sample: This involves dividing the population into distinct subgroups according to some important characteristic, such as age or socioeconomic status, and selecting a random sample out of each subgroup. If the proportion of the sample drawn from each of the subgroups, or strata, is the same as the proportion of the total population contained in each stratum (e.g., age group 40–59 constitutes 20% of the population, and 20% of the sample comes from this age stratum), then all strata will be fairly represented with regard to numbers of persons in the sample.

Systematic sample: The procedure of selecting according to some simple, systematic rule, such as all persons whose names begin with specified alphabetic letters, born on certain dates, or located at specified points on a master list. A systematic sample may lead to errors that invalidate generalizations. For example, persons' names more often begin with certain letters of the alphabet than with other letters, e.g., q, x. A systematic alphabetical sample is therefore likely to be biased.

SAMPLE, EPSEM ("equal probability of selection method") A sample selected in such a manner that all the population units have the same probability of selection. A simple random sample is an Epsem sample; a stratified sample is not unless the probability of selection is the same for all strata.

SAMPLING The process of selecting a number of subjects from all the subjects in a particular group or "universe." Conclusions based on sample results may be attributed only to the population sampled. Any extrapolation to a larger or different population is a judgment or a guess and is not part of statistical inference.

SAMPLING ERROR See ERROR.

SAMPLING VARIATION Since the inclusion of individuals in a sample is determined by chance, the results of analysis in two or more samples will differ, purely by chance. This is known as "sampling variation."

SANITARY CORDON See CORDON SANITAIRE.

SCATTER DIAGRAM (Syn: scattergram) A graphic method of displaying the distribution of two variables in relation to each other. The values for one variable are measured on the horizontal axis and the values for the other on the vertical axis.

SCENARIO BUILDING A method of predicting the future that relies on a series of assumptions about alternative possibilities, rather than on simple extrapolation of existing trends. Trend lines for demographic composition, morbidity and mortality rates, etc., can then be modified by allowing for each assumption in turn, or combinations of assumptions. The method is claimed to lead to greater flexibility in long-range health planning than simple forecasting that relies only upon extrapolation of trends.

SCREENING Screening was defined in 1951 by the US Commission on Chronic Illness as, "The presumptive identification of unrecognized disease or defect by the application of tests, examinations or other procedures which can be applied rapidly. Screening tests sort out apparently well persons who probably have a disease from those who probably do not. A screening test is not intended to be diagnostic. Persons with positive or suspicious findings must be referred to their physicians for diagnosis and necessary treatment."

Screening is an initial examination only, and positive responders require a second, diagnostic examination. The initiative for screening usually comes from the investigator or the person or agency providing care rather than from a patient with a complaint. Screening is usually concerned with chronic illness and aims to detect disease not yet under medical care.

There are different types of medical screening, each with its own aim: mass, multiple or multiphasic, and prescriptive.

Mass screening simply means the screening of a whole population.

Multiple or multiphasic screening involves the use of a variety of screening tests on the same occasion.

Prescriptive screening has as its aim the early detection in presumptively healthy individuals of disease that can be controlled better if detected early in its natural history.

The characteristics of a screening test include accuracy, estimates of yield, precision, reproducibility, sensitivity and specificity, and validity. See entries under these headings.

SCREENING LEVEL The normal limit or cutoff point at which a screening test is regarded as positive.

SEASONAL VARIATION Change in physiological status or in disease occurrence that conforms to a regular seasonal pattern.

SECONDARY ATTACK RATE The proportion of contacts who get a communicable disease as a consequence of contact with a case. The secondary attack rate is a measure of contagiousness and is useful in evaluating control measures. See also ATTACK RATE.

SECULAR TREND (Syn: temporal trend) Changes over a long period of time, generally years or decades. Examples include the decline of tuberculosis mortality and the rise, followed by a decline, in coronary heart disease mortality in the United States and many other countries in the past 50 years.

SELECTION In genetics, the force that brings about changes in the frequency of alleles and genotypes in populations through differential reproduction. In epidemiology, the process and procedure for choosing individuals for study, usually by an orderly means such as random allocation.

SELECTION BIAS See BIAS.

SEMMELWEIS, IGNAZ PHILIPP (1818–1865) An Austro-Hungarian physician-obstetrician, who discovered the cause of puerperal fever by carefully comparing infection rates in two wards of the *Allgemeines Krankenhaus* in Vienna. In one ward students customarily came direct from the mortuary or the dissecting room to the patients' bedside whereas in the other, they did not. Puerperal infection death rates were much greater in the former. Semmelweis concluded that some morbid factor was thus transmitted to women in the worse-affected ward. Unhappily, his conclusions were rejected by his colleagues.

SENSITIVITY AND SPECIFICITY (of a screening test) *Sensitivity* is the proportion of truly diseased persons in the screened population who are identified as diseased by the screening test. Sensitivity is a measure of the probability of correctly diagnosing a case, or the probability that any given case will be identified by the test (Syn: true positive rate).

Specificity is the proportion of truly nondiseased persons who are so identified by the screening test. It is a measure of the probability of correctly identifying a nondiseased person with a screening test (Syn: true negative rate). The relationships are shown in the following fourfold table, in which the letters *a, b, c,* and *d* represent the quantities specified below the table.

Screening test results	True status		Total
	Diseased	Not diseased	
Positive	a	b	$a+b$
Negative	c	d	$c+d$
Total	$a+c$	$b+d$	$a+b+c+d$

a. Diseased individuals detected by the test (true positives)
b. Nondiseased individuals positive by the test (false positives)
c. Diseased individuals not detectable by the test (false negatives)
d. Nondiseased individuals negative by the test (true negatives)

$$\text{Sensitivity} = \frac{a}{a+c} \qquad \text{Specificity} = \frac{d}{b+d}$$

$$\text{Predictive value (positive test result)} = \frac{a}{a+b}$$

$$\text{Predictive value (negative test result)} = \frac{d}{c+d}$$

See also YOUDEN'S TEST.

SENSITIVITY TESTING A study of how the final outcome of an analysis changes as a function of varying one or more of the input parameters in a prescribed manner.

SENTINEL HEALTH EVENT A condition that can be used to assess the stability or change in health levels of a population, usually by monitoring mortality statistics. Thus, death due to acute head injury is a sentinel event for a class of severe traffic injury that may be reduced by such preventive measures as use of seatbelts and crash helmets.

SENTINEL PHYSICIAN, SENTINEL PRACTICE In family medicine, a physician, practice, that undertakes to maintain surveillance for and report certain specific predetermined events, such as cases of certain communicable diseases, adverse drug reactions.

SEQUENTIAL ANALYSIS A statistical method that allows an experiment to be ended as soon as an answer of the desired precision is obtained. Study and control subjects are randomly allocated in pairs or blocks. The result of the comparison of each pair of subjects, one treated and one control, is examined as soon as it becomes available and is added to all previous results.

SERENDIPITY The accidental (and happy) discovery of important new information. A well-known example is Fleming's discovery of the bacteriocidal properties of penicillin mould. In case-control studies aimed at testing a specific hypothesis, e.g., about the relationship between tobacco and cancer, questions on other aspects of life-style have serendipitously revealed statistically significant associations, e.g., between alcohol consumption and certain cancers.

SEROEPIDEMIOLOGY Epidemiologic study or activity based on the detection on serological testing of characteristic change in the serum level of specific antibodies. Latent, subclinical infections and carrier states can thus be detected, in addition to clinically overt cases.

SEX RATIO The ratio of one sex to the other. Usually defined as the ratio of males to females (or of the rates observed in males and females).

"SHOE-LEATHER" EPIDEMIOLOGY Gathering information for epidemiologic studies by direct inquiry among the people, e.g., walking from door to door and asking questions of every householder (wearing out shoe leather in the process). JOHN SNOW did this when investigating the sources of water supply to households in the cholera epidemic in London in 1854; the method has been successfully used in many subsequent epidemic investigations. It is especially useful in investigations of sexually transmitted diseases.

SIBLINGS Children borne by the same mother.

SIBSHIP All the brothers and sisters borne by the same mother.

SICKNESS See DISEASE.

SIDE EFFECT An effect, other than the intended one, produced by a preventive, diagnostic, or therapeutic procedure or regimen.

SIGNAL-TO-NOISE RATIO A jargon term for the relationship of pertinent findings to that which is extraneous or irrelevant, or intrudes because measurement methods or other procedures are insufficiently sensitive.

SIGNIFICANCE See STATISTICAL SIGNIFICANCE.

SIMPSON'S PARADOX A form of confounding, in which the presence of a confounding variable changes the direction of an association. Simpson's paradox can occur in meta-analysis, because the sum of the data or results from a number of different studies may be affected by confounding variables that have been excluded by design features from some studies but not others; if this is not recognized, meta-analysis will be flawed. Rothman[1] has pointed out that Simpson's paradox is not really a paradox but the logical consequence of failing to recognize the presence of confounding variables.

[1] Rothman KJ: A pictorial representation of confounding in epidemiologic studies. *J Chron Dis* 28:101–108, 1975.

SIMULATION The use of a model system, e.g., a mathematical model or an animal model, to approximate the action of a real system, often used to study the properties of a real system.

SITUATION ANALYSIS Study of a situation that may require improvement. This begins with a definition of the problem, and an assessment or measurement of its extent, severity, causes, and impacts upon the community, and is followed by appraisal of interactions between the system and its environment and evaluations of performance.

SKEW DISTRIBUTION An older and less recommended term for an asymmetrical frequency distribution. If a unimodal distribution has a longer tail extending toward lower values of the variate, it is said to have negative skewness; in the contrary case, positive skewness. See also LOG-NORMAL DISTRIBUTION.

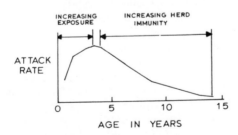

Skew distribution of attack rate of measles in relation to age.
From Lilienfeld and Lilienfeld, 1979.

SLOW VIRUS Agent causing degenerative (neurological) diseases characterized by a long incubation period and a prolonged, slowly progressive course. The best-known confirmed slow virus diseases are Creutzfeldt–Jakob disease and kuru. Multiple sclerosis is possibly a slow virus disease. Some cases of AIDS behave as slow virus disease.

Snow, John (1813–1858) London general practitioner and early anesthetist (he assisted Queen Victoria's delivery of two of her children with chloroform). His fame rests upon his observations, brilliant deductions, painstaking personal enquiries, and analytic studies of cholera outbreaks in the mid-19th century in London and elsewhere. All are recorded in *On the Mode of Communication of Cholera* (London: Churchill, 2nd ed., 1855), which can be regarded as the first definitive working text on epidemiology and which also contained an explicit statement of the germ theory of transmission, written 30 years before Koch discovered the cholera vibrio. See also NATURAL EXPERIMENT.

SOCIAL CLASS A stratum in society composed of individuals and families of equal standing. See also SOCIOECONOMIC CLASSIFICATION.

SOCIAL DRIFT Downward social class mobility as a result of impaired health often due to mental disorders.

SOCIAL MEDICINE The practice of medicine concerned with health and disease as a function of group living. Social medicine is concerned with the health of people in relation to their behavior in social groups and as such involves care of the individual patient as a member of a family and of other significant groups in everyday life. It is also concerned with the health of these groups as such and with that of the whole community as a community. See also COMMUNITY MEDICINE; PUBLIC HEALTH.

SOCIOECONOMIC CLASSIFICATION Arrangement of persons into groups according to such characteristics as prior education, occupation, and income. This usually reveals upon analysis a strong correlation with health-related characteristics such as average length of life and risk of dying from certain specific causes.

The oldest such classification that is epidemiologically useful is the Registrar-General's (RG's) occupational classification, developed in 1911 by Stephenson, Registrar-General of England and Wales. This classified all occupations into five groups—the five "social classes." Social class III is often further subdivided into nonmanual and manual groups:

    I Professional occupations
    II Intermediate occupations
    IIIN Nonmanual skilled occupations
    IIIM Manual skilled occupations
    IV Partly skilled occupations
    V Unskilled occupations

This has proven to be a valuable epidemiologic tool; social class is an accurate, consistent predictor of health experience.

There have been several other attempts to develop a more refined classification; however, most refinements require collection of more detailed information. For example, Hollingshead's scale requires details about education and income as well as occupation, and so is more time-consuming, more likely to be incomplete, and requires more costly analysis than the RG's classification. In developing countries, where up to 90% of the population may be classified under "agriculturalist" or "pastoralist" (farming or herding), other types of classifications have been developed.

One's prestige in society, and attitudes or values, e.g., setting a high value on getting a good education, are generally an integral part of social class or socioeconomic status. Attitudes toward health are often part of the set of values and may explain part of the observed difference in health between social classes.

SOCIOECONOMIC STATUS (SES) Descriptive term for a person's position in society, which may be expressed on an ORDINAL SCALE using such criteria as income, educational level attained, occupation, value of dwelling place, etc.

SOFTWARE See COMPUTER.

SOUNDEX CODE A sequence of letters used for recording names phonetically, especially in RECORD LINKAGE.

SOURCE OF INFECTION The person, animal, object, or substance from which an infectious agent passes to a host. Source of infection should be clearly distinguished from source of contamination, such as overflow of a septic tank contaminating a water supply, or an infected cook contaminating a salad. (See RESERVOIR.)[1]

[1] From *Control of Communicable Disease in Man,* 14th ed. Washington DC: American Public Health Association, 1985.

SPEARMAN'S RANK CORRELATION See CORRELATION COEFFICIENT.

SPECIFICATION

1. The process of selecting a particular functional form or model for the relationships to be analyzed in a study.
2. The process of selecting variables for inclusion in the analysis of an effect or association. This process leads to the identification of MODERATOR VARIABLES and CONFOUNDING VARIABLES. See also STRATIFICATION.

SPECIFICITY (OR A TEST) See SENSITIVITY AND SPECIFICITY.

SPECTRUM OF DISEASE The full range of manifestations of a disease; a vague term, that can mean everything from mild or subclinical or precursor states to fulminating, florid disease, or alternatively the natural history of a disease from onset to resolution.

SPELL OF SICKNESS An episode of sickness with a well-defined onset and termination. As used in the monitoring or surveillance of disease, the spell is often defined by the duration of absence from work or school.

SPLEEN RATE A term used in malaria epidemiology, to define the frequency of enlarged spleens detected on survey of a population in which malaria is prevalent. In association with the HACKETT SPLEEN CLASSIFICATION it summarizes the severity of malaria endemicity.

SPORADIC Occurring irregularly, haphazardly from time to time, and generally infrequently, e.g., cases of certain infectious diseases.

SPOT MAP Map showing the geographic location of people with a specific attribute, e.g., cases of a disease or elderly persons living alone. The making of a spot map is a common procedure in the investigation of a localized outbreak of disease. Inferences from such a map depend on the assumption that the population at risk of developing the disease is fairly evenly distributed over the area, or that at least the heterogeneities are known and can be considered in interpreting the map.

STABLE POPULATION A population that has constant fertility and mortality rates, no migration, and consequently a fixed age distribution and constant growth rate. See also STATIONARY POPULATION.

STANDARD Something that serves as a basis for comparison; a technical specification or written report drawn up by experts based on the consolidated results of scientific study, technology, and experience, aimed at optimum benefits and approved by a recognized and representative body.

STANDARD DEVIATION A measure of dispersion or variation. It is the most widely used measure of dispersion of a frequency distribution. It is equal to the positive square ROOT OF THE VARIANCE. The mean tells where the values for a group are centered. The standard deviation is a summary of how widely dispersed the values are around this center.

STANDARD ERROR The standard deviation of an estimate.

STANDARDIZATION A set of techniques used to remove as far as possible the effects of differences in age or other confounding variables, when comparing two or more populations. The common method uses weighted averaging of rates specific for age, sex, or some other potential confounding variable(s) according to some specified distribution of these variables. There are two main methods, as follows:

Direct method: The specific rates in a study population are averaged, using as weights the distribution of a specified standard population. The directly standardized rate represents what the crude rate would have been in the study population if that population had the same distribution as the standard population with respect to the variable(s) for which the adjustment or standardization was carried out.

Indirect method: This is used to compare study populations for which the specific rates are either statistically unstable or unknown. The specific rates in the standard population are averaged, using as weights the distribution of the study population. The ratio of the crude rate for the study population to the weighted average so obtained is the standardized mortality (or morbidity) ratio, or SMR. The indirectly standardized rate itself is the product of the SMR and the crude rate for the standard population.

STANDARDIZED MORTALITY (MORBIDITY) RATIO (SMR) The ratio of the number of events observed in the study group or population to the number that would be expected if the study population had the same specific rates as the standard population, multiplied by 100.

STANDARDIZED RATE RATIO (SRR) A rate ratio in which the numerator and denominator rates have been standardized to the same (standard) population distribution.

STANDARD METROPOLITAN STATISTICAL AREA Because of the extensive interactions between a city and its surrounding areas, a unit encompassing both is needed as a base for statistical description. The concept of a standard metropolitan statistical area (SMSA) was introduced in the United States to furnish such a unit. To qualify as an SMSA an area has to meet criteria related to size, social and economic integration of the city and surrounding county or counties, minimum population density, and minimum proportion of the labor force engaged in nonagricultural work.

STATIONARY POPULATION A stable population that has a zero growth rate with constant numbers of births and deaths each year.

STATISTICS The science and art of collecting, summarizing, and analyzing data that are subject to random variation. The term is also applied to the data themselves and to summarizations of the data. Statistical terms are defined by Kendall and Buckland.[1]

[1] Kendall MG, Buckland WR: *A Dictionary of Statistical Terms*, 4th ed. London: Longman, 1982.

STATISTICAL ERROR See ERROR.

STATISTICAL INFERENCE See INFERENCE.

STATISTICAL MODEL See MATHEMATICAL MODEL.

STATISTICAL SIGNIFICANCE Statistical methods allow an estimate to be made of the probability of the observed or greater degree of association between independent and dependent variables under the null hypothesis. From this estimate, in a sample of given size, the statistical "significance" of a result can be stated. Usually the level of statistical significance is stated by the P VALUE.

STATISTICAL TEST A procedure that is intended to decide whether a hypothesis about the distribution of one or more populations or variables should be rejected or accepted. Statistical tests may be parametric or nonparametric.

STEREOGRAM (Syn: isometric chart) A graph or chart that displays more than two variables in a manner that appears three-dimensional to the eye.

STOCHASTIC PROCESS A process that incorporates some element of randomness.

STRATEGY In game theory, a mathematical function.

STRATIFICATION The process of or result of separating a sample into several subsamples according to specified criteria such as age groups, socioeconomic status, etc. The effect of confounding variables may be controlled by stratifying the analysis of results. For example, lung cancer is known to be associated with smoking. To examine the possible association between urban atmospheric pollution and lung cancer, controlling for smoking, the population may be divided into strata according to smoking status. The association between air pollution and cancer can then be appraised separately within each stratum. Stratification is used not only to control for confounding effects but also as a way of detecting modifying effects. In this example, stratification makes it possible to examine the effect of smoking on the association between atmospheric pollution and lung cancer.

STRATIFIED RANDOMIZATION (Syn: blocked randomization) A randomization procedure in which strata are identified and subjects randomly allocated within each. This produces a situation intermediate between paired allocation and simple random allocation.

STUDY DESIGN See RESEARCH DESIGN.

SUBCLINICAL DISEASE See DISEASE, SUBCLINICAL.

SURVEILLANCE Ongoing scrutiny, generally using methods distinguished by their practicability, uniformity, and frequently their rapidity, rather than by complete accuracy. Its main purpose is to detect changes in trend or distribution in order to initiate investigative or control measures. See also MONITORING.

SURVEILLANCE OF DISEASE The continuing scrutiny of all aspects of occurrence and spread of a disease that are pertinent to effective control.

Included are the systematic collection and evaluation of (1) morbidity and mortality reports, (2) special reports of field investigations of epidemics and of individual cases, (3) isolation and identification of infectious agents by laboratories, (4) data concerning the availability, use, and untoward effects of vaccines and toxoids, immune globulins, insecticides, and other substances used in control, (5) information regarding immunity levels in segments of the population, and (6) other relevant epidemiologic data. A report summarizing these data should be prepared and distributed to all cooperating persons and others with a need to know the results of the surveillance activities. The procedure applies to all jurisdictional levels of public health from local to international.[1] Serological surveillance identifies patterns of current and past infection using serological test. See also SEROEPIDEMIOLOGY.

[1] Benenson AS (Ed.): *Control of Communicable Diseases in Man,* 14th ed. Washington DC: American Public Health Association, 1985.

SURVEY An investigation in which information is systematically collected but in which the experimental method is not used. A population survey may be conducted by face-to-face inquiry, by self-completed questionnaires, by telephone, postal service, or in some other way. Each method has its advantages and disadvantages. For instance, a face-to-face (interview) survey may be a better way than self-completed questionnaire to collect information on attitudes or feelings, but it is more costly. Existing medical or other records may contain accurate information, but not about a representative sample of the population.

The information that is gathered in a survey is usually complex enough to require editing (for accuracy, completeness, etc.), coding, keypunching, i.e., entry on PUNCH CARDS and processing and analysis by machine or computer. The generalizability of results depends upon the extent to which the surveyed population is representative.

The term "survey" is sometimes used in a narrow sense to refer specifically to a FIELD SURVEY.

SURVEY INSTRUMENT The interview schedule, questionnaire, medical examination record form, etc., used in a survey.

SURVIVAL ANALYSIS A class of statistical procedures for estimating the SURVIVAL FUNCTION, and for making inferences about the effects on it of treatments, prognostic factors, exposures, and other covariates.

SURVIVAL CURVE A curve that starts at 100% of the study population and shows the percentage of the population still surviving at successive times for as long as information is available. May be applied not only to survival as such, but also to the persistence of freedom from a disease, or complication or some other endpoint.

SURVIVAL FUNCTION (Syn: survival distribution) A function of time, usually denoted by $S(t)$, that starts with a population 100% well at a particular time and provides the percentage of the population still well at later times. Survival functions may be applied to any discrete event, for example, disease incidence or relapse, death, or recovery after onset of disease (in which case the population is initially 100% diseased, and the "survival" function gives the percentage still diseased).

SURVIVAL RATE (Syn: cumulative survival rate) The proportion of survivors in a group, e.g., of patients, studied and followed over a period. The proportion of persons in a specified group alive at the beginning of the time interval (e.g., a five-year period) who survive to the end of the interval. It is equal to 1 minus the CUMULATIVE MORTALITY RATE. May be studied by current or COHORT LIFE TABLE methods.

SURVIVAL RATIO The probability of surviving between one age and another; when computed for age groups, the ratios correspond to those of the person-years-lived function of a life table.

SURVIVORSHIP STUDY Use of a cohort LIFE TABLE to provide the probability that an event, such as death, will occur in successive intervals of time after diagnosis and, conversely, the probability of surviving each interval. The multiplication of these probabilities of survival for each time interval for those alive at the beginning of that interval yields a cumulative probability of surviving for the total period of study.

SYDENHAM, THOMAS (1624–1689) A great English physician in the tradition of Hippocrates and one of the founding fathers of epidemiology (although his ideas about the meteorological causes of epidemics were wrong). His writings contain many careful and comprehensive accounts of important epidemic diseases, notably plague, malaria, measles, dysentery, and scarlet fever. His *Opera Omni* have been twice translated into English; the second (and better) two-volume translation by Latham was published by the Sydenham Society in 1848–1850.

SYMBIOSIS The biological association of two or more species to their mutual benefit.

SYMMETRICAL RELATIONSHIP An association between variables that does not have direction.

The following four varieties can be distinguished:

1. Functional interdependence, where one variable cannot exist without the other; e.g., prevalence is a function of incidence and duration.
2. Common complex, where variables occur together without being interdependent or necessary to each other; e.g., the occurrence together of air pollution, poverty, poor housing, and overcrowding.
3. Alternative indicators of the same entity; e.g., antibodies to a microorganism and history of specific infection caused by that microorganism.
4. The effects of a common cause; e.g., clinical and biochemical changes in hepatitis.

See also ASSOCIATION, SYMMETRICAL.

SYNDROME A symptom complex in which the symptoms and/or signs coexist more frequently than would be expected by chance on the assumption of independence.

SYNERGISM, SYNERGY The definition of synergism in epidemiology is somewhat controversial. We offer two definitions, the first a common dictionary definition, the second a more specific definition encountered in bioassay.

1. A situation in which the combined effect of two or more factors is greater than the sum of their solitary effects.
2. Two factors act synergistically if there are persons who will get the disease when exposed to both factors but not when exposed to either alone. ANTAGONISM, the opposite of synergism, exists if there are persons who will get the disease when exposed to one of the factors alone, but not when exposed to both. Note that under these definitions two factors may act synergistically in some persons and antagonistically in others.

SYSTEMATIC ERROR See BIAS.

SYSTEMS ANALYSIS This term is used with three similar meanings:

1. The examination of various elements of a system with a view to ascertaining whether the proposed solution to a problem will fit into the system and, in turn, effect an overall improvement in the system.
2. The analysis of an activity in order to determine precisely what is required of the system, how this can best be accomplished, and in what ways the computer can be useful.
3. Systems analysis refers to any formal analysis whose purpose is to suggest a course of action by systematically examining the objectives, costs, effectiveness and risks of alternative policies or strategies and designing additional ones if those examined are found wanting. It is an approach to or way of looking at complex problems of choice under uncertainty; it is not yet a method.

T

TAKAKI, KANEHIRO (1849–1915) Japanese nobleman who studied medicine at St Thomas's Hospital Medical School, London. He became a naval surgeon, and later used his opportunity as director of naval medical services to conduct large-scale dietary experiments on populations of naval personnel, demonstrating that beriberi could be prevented by a mixed diet containing protein as well as rice.

TARGET POPULATION
1. The collection of individuals, items, measurements, etc., about which we want to make inferences. The term is sometimes used to indicate the population from which a sample is drawn and sometimes to denote any "reference" population about which inferences are required.
2. The group of persons for whom an intervention is planned.

TAXONOMY A systematic classification into related groups.

TAXONOMY OF DISEASE The orderly classification of diseases into appropriate categories on the basis of relationships among them, with the application of names. See also NOSOGRAPHY, NOSOLOGY.

t-DISTRIBUTION, t-TEST The t-distribution is the distribution of a quotient of independent random variables, the numerator of which is a standardized normal variate and the denominator of which is the positive square root of the quotient of a chi-square distributed variate and its number of degrees of freedom. The t-test uses a statistic that, under the null hypothesis, has the t-distribution, to test whether two means differ significantly, or to test linear regression or correlation coefficients. The t-distribution and the t-test were developed by WS Gossett, who wrote under the pseudonym "Student" as his employment precluded individual publication.

TERATOGEN A substance that produces abnormalities in the embryo or fetus by disturbing maternal homeostasis or by acting directly on the fetus in utero.

TEST OF SIGNIFICANCE See P VALUE; STATISTICAL SIGNIFICANCE.

TEST HYPOTHESIS See NULL HYPOTHESIS.

THEORETICAL EPIDEMIOLOGY The development of mathematical/statistical models to explain different aspects of the occurrence of a variety of diseases. With some infectious diseases, models have been generated to elucidate the reasons for epidemics and/or to predict the behavior of the disease in reaction to given control measures. See also MODEL.

THERAPEUTIC TRIAL See CLINICAL TRIAL.

THRESHHOLD LIMIT VALUE See SAFETY STANDARDS.

THRESHOLD PHENOMENA Events or changes that occur only after a certain level of a characteristic is reached.

TIME CLUSTER See CLUSTERING.

TIME–PLACE CLUSTER See CLUSTERING.

TOTAL FERTILITY RATE (TFR) The average number of children that would be born per woman if all women lived to the end of their childbearing years and bore children according to a given set of age-specific fertility rates. It is computed by summing the age-specific fertility rates for all ages and multiplying by the interval into which the ages are grouped. The TFR is an important fertility measure, providing the most accurate answer to the question, "How many children does a women have, on average?"

TRACER DISEASE METHOD Tracer or indicator conditions as defined by Kessner[1] are easily diagnosed, reasonably frequent illnesses or health states whose outcomes are believed to be affected by health care and which taken in aggregate should reflect the gamut of patients and health problems encountered in a medical practice. The extent to which the recorded care of these conditions concurs with preset standards of care is used as an index of the quality of care delivered. However, it should first be shown that the preset standards contribute to a favorable outcome. See also SENTINEL HEALTH EVENT.

[1] Kessner DM, Snow CK, Singer J: *Assessment of Medical Care for Children.* Washington DC: National Academy of Sciences, Institute of Medicine, 1974.

TRANSMISSION OF INFECTION Transmission of infectious agents. Any mechanism by which an infectious agent is spread through the environment or to another person. These mechanisms are defined in *Control of Communicable Disease in Man*[1] as follows:

    a. Direct transmission

        Direct and essentially immediate transfer of infectious agents (other than from an arthropod in which the organism has undergone essential multiplication or development) to a receptive portal of entry through which human infection may take place. This may be by direct contract as by touching, kissing, or sexual intercourse, or by the direct projection (droplet spread) of droplet spray onto the conjunctiva or onto the mucous membranes of the nose or mouth during sneezing, coughing, spitting, singing, or talking (usually limited to a distance of about 1 m or less). It may also be by direct exposure of susceptible tissue to an agent in soil, compost, or decaying vegetable matter in which it normally leads a saprophytic existence, (e.g., the systemic mycoses), or by the bite of a rabid animal. Transplacental transmission is another form of direct transmission.

    b. Indirect transmission

        Vehicle-borne—Contaminated materials or objects (fomites) such as toys, handkerchiefs, soiled clothes, bedding, cooking or eating utensils, and surgical instruments or dressings (indirect contact); water, food, milk, biological products including blood, serum, plasma, tissues, or organs; or any substance serving as an intermediate means by which an infectious agent is transported and introduced into a susceptible host through a suitable portal of entry. The agent may or may not have multiplied or developed in or on the vehicle before being transmitted.

        Vector-borne—(1) *Mechanical:* Includes simple mechanical carriage by a crawling or flying insect through soiling of its feet or proboscis, or by passage of organisms through its gastrointestinal tract. This does not require multiplication or development of the organism. (2) *Biological:* Propagation (multiplication), cyclic development, or a combination of these (cyclopropagative) is required before the arthropod can transmit the infective form of the agent to man. An incubation period (extrinsic) is required following infection before the arthropod becomes infective. The infectious agent may be passed vertically to succeeding generations (transovarian transmission); transstadial transmission is its passage from the one stage of the life cycle to another, as nymph to adult. Transmission may be by saliva during biting or by regurgitation or deposition on the skin of feces or other material capable of penetrating subsequently through the bite wound or through an area of trauma from scratching or rubbing. This is transmission by an infected nonvertebrate host and must be differentiated for epidemiologic purposes from simple mechanical carriage by a vector in the role of a vehicle. An arthropod in either role is termed a "vector."

Airborne—The dissemination of microbial aerosols to a suitable portal of entry, usually the respiratory tract. Microbial aerosols are suspensions in the air of particles consisting partially or wholly of microorganisms. Particles in the $1-5\mu$ range are easily drawn into the alveoli of the lungs and may be retained there; many are exhaled from the alveoli without deposition. They may remain suspended in the air for long periods of time, some retaining and others losing infectivity or virulence. Not considered as airborne are droplets and other large particles that promptly settle out (see Direct transmission, above).

The following are airborne and their mode of transmission is direct:

Droplet nuclei: Usually the small residues that result from evaporation of fluid from droplets emitted by an infected host (see above). Droplet nuclei also may be created purposely by a variety of atomizing devices, or accidentally as in microbiology laboratories or in abattoirs, rendering plants, or autopsy rooms. They usually remain suspended in the air for long periods of time.

Dust: The small particles of widely varying size that may arise from soil (as, for example, fungus spores separated from dry soil by wind or mechanical agitation), clothes, bedding, or contaminated floors.[1] See also ACQUAINTANCE NETWORK; AIR-BORNE INFECTION; CARRIER; COMMON VEHICLE SPREAD; CONTACT; CONTAMINATION; DROPLET NUCLEI.

[1] Benenson AS (Ed.): *Control of Communicable Diseases in Man,* 14th ed. Washington DC: American Public Health Association, 1985.

TRANSOVARIAL TRANSMISSION See VECTOR-BORNE INFECTION.

TRANSPORT HOST See PARATENIC HOST.

TREND A long-term movement in an ordered series, e.g., a time series. An essential feature is that the movement, while possibly irregular in the short term, shows movement consistently in the same direction over a long term. The term is also used loosely to refer to an association which is consistent in several samples or strata but is not statistically significant.

TREND LINE That line that best fits the distribution of a set of values plotted on two axes.

TRIAL See CLINICAL TRIAL.

TROHOC STUDY A retrospective case-control study. The term, proposed by AR Feinstein,[1] is the inversion of "cohort;" its use is deprecated by the great majority of epidemiologists.

[1] *Clin Pharmacol Ther* 30:564–577, 1981.

TYPE I ERROR See ERROR.

TYPE II ERROR See ERROR.

TWIN STUDY Method of detecting genetic etiology in human disease. The basic premise of twin studies is that monozygotic twins, being formed by the division of a single fertilized ovum, carry identical genes, while dizygotic twins, being formed by the fertilization of two ova by two different spermatozoa, are genetically no more similar than two siblings born after separate pregnancies.

TWO-TAIL TEST A statistical significance test based on the assumption that the data are distributed in both directions from some central value(s).

U, V

UNBIASSED ESTIMATOR An estimator that for all sample sizes has an expected value equal to the parameter being estimated. If an estimator tends to be unbiassed as sample size increases, it is referred to as asymptotically unbiassed.

UNDERLYING CAUSE OF DEATH See DEATH CERTIFICATE.

UNDERREPORTING Failure to identify and/or count all cases, leading to reduction of numerator in a rate. See also ERROR.

UTILITY In economics, this means satisfaction derived from obtaining some quantity of a specified article of commerce. When used in decision theory or CLINICAL DECISION ANALYSIS, the meaning is essentially the same, and can be expressed as the usefulness or desirability of an outcome resulting from a decision.

VACCINATION Strictly speaking, vaccination refers to inoculation (from Latin *in oculus,* into a bud) with vaccinia virus against smallpox. Nowadays the word is broadly used synonymously with procedures for immunization against all infectious disease.

VACCINE Immunobiological substance used for active immunization by introducing into the body a live modified, attenuated, or killed inactivated infectious organism or its toxin. The vaccine is capable of stimulating immune response by the host, who is thus rendered resistant to infection. The word "vaccine" was originally applied to the serum from a cow infected with vaccinia virus (cowpox; from Latin *vacca,* cow); it is now used of all immunizing agents.

VALIDATION The process of establishing that a method is sound.

VALIDITY This term, derived from the Latin *validus,* strong, has several meanings, usually accompanied by a qualifying word or phrase.

VALIDITY, MEASUREMENT An expression of the degree to which a measurement measures what it purports to measure.

Several varieties are distinguished, including construct validity, content validity, and criterion validity (concurrent and predictive validity).

Construct validity: The extent to which the measurement corresponds to theoretical concepts (constructs) concerning the phenomenon under study. For example, if on theoretical grounds, the phenomenon should change with age, a measurement with construct validity would reflect such a change.

Content validity: The extent to which the measurement incorporates the domain of the phenomenon under study. For example, a measurement of functional health status should embrace activities of daily living, occupational, family, and social functioning, etc.

Criterion validity: The extent to which the measurement correlates with an external criterion of the phenomenon under study. Two aspects of criterion validity can be distinguished:

1. *Concurrent validity:* The measurement and the criterion refer to the same point in time. An example would be a visual inspection of a wound for evidence of

infection validated against bacteriological examination of a specimen taken at the same time.

2. *Predictive validity:* The measurement's validity is expressed in terms of its ability to predict the criterion. An example would be an academic aptitude test that was validated against subsequent academic performance.

VALIDITY, STUDY The degree to which the inference drawn from a study, especially generalizations extending beyond the study sample, are warranted when account is taken of the study methods, the representativeness of the study sample, and the nature of the population from which it is drawn. Two varieties of study validity are distinguished:

1. *Internal validity:* The index and comparison groups are selected and compared in such a manner that the observed differences between them on the dependent variables under study may, apart from sampling error, be attributed only to the hypothesized effect under investigation.

2. *External validity (generalizability):* A study is externally valid or generalizable if it can produce unbiased inferences regarding a target population (beyond the subjects in the study). This aspect of validity is only meaningful with regard to a specified external target population. For example, the results of a study conducted using only white male subjects might or might not be generalizable to all human males (the target population consisting of all human males). It is not generalizable to females (the target population consisting of all people). The evaluation of generalizability usually involves much more subject-matter judgment than internal validity.

These epidemiologic definitions of the terms "internal validity" and "external validity" do not correspond exactly to some definitions found in the sociological literature.

VARIABLE Any quantity that varies. Any attribute, phenomenon, or event that can have different values.

VARIABLE, ANTECEDENT A variable that causally precedes the association or outcome under study. See also EXPLANATORY VARIABLE; INDEPENDENT VARIABLE.

VARIABLE, CONFOUNDING See CONFOUNDING.

VARIABLE, CONTROL Independent variable other than the "hypothetical causal variable" that has a potential effect on the dependent variable and is subject to control by analysis.

VARIABLE, DEPENDENT See DEPENDENT VARIABLE.

VARIABLE, DISTORTER A CONFOUNDING VARIABLE that diminishes, masks, or reverses the association under study.

VARIABLE, EXPERIENTIAL See INDEPENDENT VARIABLE.

VARIABLE INDEPENDENT See INDEPENDENT VARIABLE.

VARIABLE, INTERVENING See INTERVENING VARIABLE.

VARIABLE, MANIFESTATIONAL See DEPENDENT VARIABLE.

VARIABLE, MODERATOR See EFFECT MODIFIER.

VARIABLE, PASSENGER See PASSENGER VARIABLE.

VARIABLE, UNCONTROLLED A (potentially) confounding variable that has not been brought under control by design or analysis. See also CONFOUNDING.

VARIANCE A measure of the variation shown by a set of observations, defined by the sum of the squares of deviations from the mean, divided by the number of DEGREES OF FREEDOM in the set of observations.

VARIATE (Syn: random variable) A variable that may assume any of a set of values, each with a preassigned probability (known as its distribution).

VECTOR

1. In infectious disease epidemiology, an insect or any living carrier that transports an infectious agent from an infected individual or its wastes to a susceptible individual or its food or immediate surroundings. The organism may or may not pass through a developmental cycle within the vector.

2. In statistics, an ordered set of numbers representing the values of a set of variables.

VECTOR-BORNE INFECTION Several classes of vector-borne infections are recognized, each with epidemiologic features that are determined by the interaction between the infectious agent and the human host, on the one hand, and the vector on the other. Therefore, environmental factors such as climatic and seasonal variations influence the epidemiologic pattern by virtue of their effects on the vector and its habits.

The terms used to describe specific features of vector-borne infections are:

Biological transmission: Transmission of the infectious agent to susceptible host by bite of blood-feeding (arthropod) vector as in malaria, or by other inoculation, as in *Schistosoma* infection.

Extrinsic incubation period: Time necessary after acquisition of infection by the (arthropod) vector for the infectious agent to multiply or develop sufficiently so that it can be transmitted by the vector to a vertebrate host.

Hibernation: A possible mechanism by which the infected vector survives adverse cold weather by becoming dormant.

Inapparent infection: Response to infection without developing overt signs of illness. If this is accompanied by viremia or bacteremia in a high proportion of infected animals or persons, the receptor species is well suited as an epidemiologically important host in the transmission cycle.

Mechanical transmission: Transport of the infectious agent between hosts by arthropod vectors with contaminated mouthparts, antennae, or limbs. There is no multiplication of the infectious agent in the vector.

Overwintering: Persistence of the infectious microorganism in the vector for extended periods, such as the cooler winter months, during which the vector has no opportunity to be reinfected or to infect a vertebrate host. Overwintering is an important concept in the epidemiology of vector-borne diseases since the annual recrudescence of viral activity after periods (winter, dry season) adverse to continual transmission depends upon a mechanism for local survival of an infectious microorganism or its reintroduction from outside the endemic area. To some extent, the risk of a summertime epidemic may be determined by the relative success of microorganism survival in the local winter reservoir. Since overwinter survival may in turn depend upon the level of activity of the microorganism during the preceding summer–fall, outbreaks sometimes occur for two or more successive years.

Transovarial infection (transmission): Transmission of the infectious microorganism from the affected female arthropod to her progeny.

VECTOR SPACE An area (or volume) defined by the specified dimensions of two (or three) vectors.

VEHICLE OF INFECTION TRANSMISSION The mode of transmission of an infectious agent from its reservoir to a susceptible host. This can be person-to-person, food, vector-borne, etc.

VENN DIAGRAM A pictorial presentation of the extent to which two or more quantities or concepts are mutually inclusive and mutually exclusive.

VIRCHOW, RUDOLF (1821–1902) Born in Pomerania, Virchow graduated in medicine from Berlin in 1843 and rapidly established his reputation as the leading medical

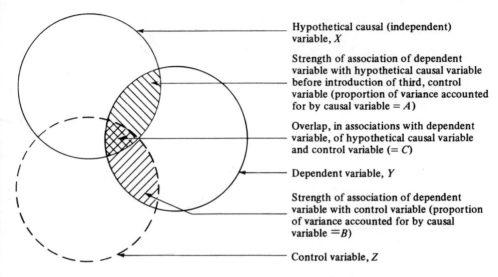

Hypothetical causal (independent) variable, *X*

Strength of association of dependent variable with hypothetical causal variable before introduction of third, control variable (proportion of variance accounted for by causal variable $= A$)

Overlap, in associations with dependent variable, of hypothetical causal variable and control variable ($= C$)

Dependent variable, *Y*

Strength of association of dependent variable with control variable (proportion of variance accounted for by causal variable $= B$)

Control variable, *Z*

Venn diagram. *From* Susser, 1973.

scientist of his time. Modern pathology owes much to his rigorous use of hypothesis-testing methods, illustrated in his first paper in the journal he founded, *Archiv für pathologische Anatomie*, now universally known as Virchow's Archives. Virchow was also a practicing epidemiologist, who investigated a serious epidemic of typhus in Silesia in 1848; his recommendations for hygienic and social reform got him into trouble with the government, but his scientific brilliance made it impossible for the authorities not to recognize and reward him with promotions and honors. He entered Parliament in 1862, and during the Franco-Prussian War he organized an ambulance service. He made many contributions of fundamental importance to the science of pathology, but deserves to be remembered as a great humanitarian as well.

VIRGIN POPULATION A population that has never been exposed to a particular infectious agent.

VIRULENCE The degree of pathogenicity; the disease-evoking power of a microorganism in a given host. Numerically expressed as the ratio of the number of cases of overt infection in the total number infected, as determined by immunoassay. When death is the only criterion of severity, this is the case-fatality rate.

VITAL RECORDS (Literally, "To do with living") Certificates of birth, death, marriage, and divorce required for legal and demographic purposes.

VITAL STATISTICS Systematically tabulated information concerning births, marriages, divorces, separations, and deaths based on registrations of these vital events.

W, X, Y, Z

WASHOUT PHASE That stage in a study, especially a therapeutic trial, when treatment is withdrawn so that its effects disappear and the subject's characteristics return to their baseline state.

WORM COUNT A method of surveillance of helminth infection of the gut that depends upon counts of worms, or their cysts or ova, in quantitatively titrated samples of feces. Other terms used to describe this form of surveillance are "egg count," "cyst count," and "parasite count."

WU, LIEN-TEH (1879–1960) Chinese epidemiologist, responsible for controlling the plague pandemic in Manchuria in 1910–11. Later he worked on control of sexually transmitted diseases and other socioeconomically determined health conditions, developed a national quarantine service and was one of the founders of the Chinese Medical Association, thus helping to lay the foundations for health improvements in modern China.

XENOBIOTIC

1. (Syn: commensal, symbiosis) Pertaining to association of two animal species, usually insects, in the absence of a dependency relationship, as opposed to parasitism.
2. A foreign compound that is metabolized in the body. Many pesticides and their derivatives, some food additives and a number of other complex organic compounds such as dioxins and PCBs, are xenobiotics.

XENODIAGNOSIS Detection of a (human) pathogenic organism by allowing a noninfected vector (e.g., mosquito) to consume infected material, and then examining this vector for evidence of the pathogen.

YATES' CORRECTION An adjustment proposed by Yates (1934) in the chi-square calculation for a 2×2 table, which brings the distribution based on discontinuous frequencies closer to the continuous chi-square distribution from which the published tables for testing chi-squares are derived

YEARS OF POTENTIAL LIFE LOST (YPLL) See POTENTIAL YEARS OF LIFE LOST.

YIELD The number or proportion of cases of a condition accurately identified by a screening test.

YOUDEN'S INDEX When assessing screening tests, in the uncommon case where the risk of a false negative and that of a false positive result are assumed to be equivalent (i.e., specificity and sensitivity assumed to be equally important), it may be possible to compare screening tests through the Youden index based on the sum of specificity and sensitivity:

$$\text{Youden Index} = J = \text{specificity} + \text{sensitive} - 1$$

with J ranging from zero (specificity $= 0.50$ and sensitivity $= 0.50$) to 1 (sensitivity $= 1.00$, specificity $= 1.00$).

ZERO-TIME SHIFT This concerns the selection of a starting point for the measurement of survival following the detection of disease. It is a jargon term, denoting the movement "backward" (toward the starting point of a disease) of time between onset and detection, that may accompany use of a screening procedure.

ZOONOSIS An infection or infectious disease transmissible under natural conditions from vertebrate animals to man. Examples include rabies and plague. May be enzootic or epizootic.

Bibliography

Many of the works on this list contain glossaries, and nearly all contain definitions that have been adapted and included in this dictionary.

Abramson JH: *Survey Methods in Community Medicine*, 3rd ed. London: Churchill Livingstone, 1984.

Alderson M: *An Introduction to Epidemiology*, 2nd ed. London: Macmillan, 1983.

Allaby M: *Dictionary of the Environment*. Southampton: London Press, 1975.

Armitage P: *Statistical Methods in Medical Research*. Oxford: Blackwell, 1971.

Bahn AK: *Basic Medical Statistics*. New York: Grune & Stratton, 1972.

Barker DJP, Rose G: *Epidemiology in Medical Practice*, 2nd ed. Edinburgh: Churchill Livingstone, 1979.

Benenson AS (Ed): *Control of Communicable Diseases in Man*, 14th ed. Washington DC: American Public Health Association, 1985.

Bogue DJ: *Principles of Demography*. New York: Wiley, 1969.

Breslow NE, Day NE: *Statistical Methods in Cancer Research, Vol 1: The Analysis of Case-Control Data*. Lyon: IARC, 1980.

Cavalli-Sforza LL, Bodmer WF: *The Genetics of Human Populations*. San Francisco: Freeman, 1971.

Colton T: *Statistics in Medicine*. Boston: Little, Brown, 1974.

Committee on Population and Demography, National Academy of Science/National Research Council: *Collecting Data for the Estimation of Fertility and Mortality*. Washington DC: National Academy Press, Report Number 6, 1981.

Cox DR, Hinkley DV: *Theoretical Statistics*. New York: Chapman and Hall, 1974.

Davies G: *A Dictionary of Veterinary Epidemiology*. Mimeographed. To be published.

Dublin LI, Lotka AJ: *The Money Value of a Man*. New York: Ronald, 1930.

Farr, W: *Vital Statistics* (Ed. NA Humphreys). London: Stanford, 1885. [A modern abridgement, edited by A Adelstein and MW Susser, was published by the New York Academy of Medicine in 1975.]

Feinstein AR: *Clinical Biostatistics*. St Louis: Mosby, 1974.

Feinstein AR: *Clinical Epidemiology*. Philadelphia: Saunders, 1985.

Feinstein AR: A glossary of neologisms in quantitative clinical science. *Clin Pharmacol Ther* 30:564–77, 1981.

Fisher RA: *Statistical Methods and Scientific Inference*. Edinburgh: Oliver and Boyd, 1956.

Fleiss JL: *Statistical Methods for Rates and Proportions*, 2nd ed. New York: Wiley, 1981.

Fletcher RH, Fletcher SW, Wagner EH: *Clinical Epidemiology—The Essentials*. Baltimore: Williams & Wilkins, 1982.

Friedman GD: *Primer of Epidemiology*, 2nd ed. New York: McGraw-Hill, 1980.

Froom J: An international glossary for primary care. *J Family Pract* 13:673–681, 1981.

Garrison FH: *An Introduction to the History of Medicine*, 4th ed. Philadelphia: Saunders, 1929.

Greenwood M: *Epidemics and Crowd Diseases.* London: Williams and Norgate, 1933.

Haupt A, Kane TT: *Population Handbook,* 2nd ed. Washington DC: Population Reference Bureau, 1985.

Hogarth J: *Glossary of Health Care Terminology.* Copenhagen: World Health Organization, 1975.

Holland WW (Ed): *Data Handling in Epidemiology.* London: Oxford, 1970.

Holland WW (Ed): *Evaluation of Health Care.* Oxford: Oxford University Press, 1983.

Holland WW, Detels R, Knox G (Eds): *Oxford Textbook of Public Health,* Vol 3. Oxford: Oxford University Press, 1985.

Ibrahim MA: *Epidemiology and Health Policy.* Rockville, MD: Aspen, 1985.

Jammal A, Allard R, Loslier G (Eds): Dictionnaire d'épidémiologie. St Hyacinthe, Maloine, Paris: Edisem, 1988.

Jenicek M, Cléroux R: *Épidémiologie.* St Hyacinthe, Québec: Edisem, 1982.

Kahn HA: *An Introduction to Epidemiologic Methods.* New York: Oxford University Press, 1983.

Kelsey JL, Thompson WD, Evans AS: *Methods in Observational Epidemiology.* New York: Oxford University Press, 1986.

Kendall MG, Buckland AA: *A Dictionary of Statistical Terms,* 4th ed. London: Longman, 1982.

Kleinbaum DG, Kupper LL, Morgenstern H: *Epidemiology—Principles and Quantitative Methods.* Belmont: Lifetime Learning Publications, 1982.

Klug WS, Cummings MR: *Concepts of Genetics.* Columbus OH: Merrill, 1986.

Knox EG (Ed): *Epidemiology in Health Care Planning.* London: Oxford University Press, 1979.

Last JM (Ed): *Maxcy-Rosenau Public Health and Preventive Medicine,* 12th ed. Norwalk, CT: Appleton-Century-Crofts, 1986.

Last JM: *Public Health and Human Ecology.* Norwalk CT: Appleton and Lange, 1987.

Lilienfeld AM, Lilienfeld D: *Foundations of Epidemiology,* 2nd ed. New York: Oxford University Press, 1979.

Macmahon B, Pugh TF: *Epidemiology: Principles and Methods.* Boston: Little, Brown, 1970.

Mausner JS, Kramer S: *Epidemiology,* 2nd ed. Philadelphia: Saunders, 1985.

McDowell I, Newell C: *Measuring Health: A Guide to Rating Scales and Questionnaires.* New York: Oxford University Press, 1987.

Meadows AJ, Gordon M, Singleton A: *Dictionary of New Information Technology.* London: Century, 1982.

Meinert CL: *Clinical Trials.* New York: Oxford University Press, 1986.

Miettinen OS: *Theoretical Epidemiology.* New York: Wiley, 1985.

Morris JN: *Uses of Epidemiology,* 3rd ed. London: Churchill Livingstone, 1975.

Morrison AS: *Screening in Chronic Disease.* New York: Oxford University Press, 1985.

Morton NE: *Outline of genetic epidemiology.* New York: Karger, 1982.

Murphy EA: *The Logic of Medicine.* Baltimore: Johns Hopkins University Press, 1976.

Murphy EA: *A Companion to Medical Statistics.* Baltimore: Johns Hopkins University Press, 1985.

Oldham PD: *Measurement in Medicine.* Baltimore: Johns Hopkins University Press, 1976.

Oxford English Dictionary (OED). London: Oxford University Press, 1971.

Pressat R: *Dictionary of Demography.* English Trans. Ed. Christopher Wilson. Oxford: Blackwell, 1985.

Rimm AA, Hartz AJ, Kalbfleisch JH, Anderson AJ, Hoffmann RG: *Basic Biostatistics in Medicine and Epidemiology.* New York: Appleton-Century-Crofts, 1980.

Rothman KJ: *Modern Epidemiology.* Boston: Little, Brown, 1986.

Rothman KJ (Ed): *Causal Inference.* Chestnut Hill, MA: Epidemiology Resources, Inc., 1988.

Rumeau-Rouquette C, Breart G, Padieu R: *Méthodes en épidémiologie.* Paris: Flammarion, 1980.

Schlesselman JJ: *Case-Control Studies; Design, Conduct, Analysis.* New York: Oxford University Press, 1982.

Schuman SH: *Practice-Based Epidemiology.* New York: Gordon and Breach, 1986.

Silverman WA: *Human Experimentation: A Guided Step into the Unknown.* Oxford: Oxford University Press, 1985.

Skinner HA: *The Origin of Medical Terms,* 2nd ed. Baltimore: Williams & Wilkins, 1961.

Snedecor GW, Cochran WH: *Statistical Methods,* 7th Ed. Ames, IO: Iowa University Press, 1979.

Snow, J: *On the Mode of Communication of Cholera,* 2nd ed. London: Churchill, 1855. [Reprinted 1936 by the Commonwealth Fund of New York, with an Introduction by Wade Hampton Frost; and again by Hafner, New York, 1973.]

Sohm ED (Ed): *Glossary of Evaluation Terms.* Geneva: United Nations, 1978.

Stalleybrass CO: *The Principles of Epidemiology.* London: Routledge, 1931.

Stedman's Medical Dictionary, 22nd ed. Baltimore: Williams & Wilkins, 1972.

Susser MW: *Causal Thinking in the Health Sciences.* New York: Oxford University Press, 1973.

Susser MW, Watson W, Hopper K: *Sociology in Medicine,* 3rd ed. New York: Oxford University Press, 1985.

Swaroop S: *Introduction to Health Statistics.* Edinburgh: Livingstone, 1960.

Toma B (Ed): Glossaire d'épidémiologie animale. Mimeographed. Ecole Nationale Veterinaire D'Alfort, 1987.

van de Walle E: *Multilingual Demographic Dictionary; English Section.* Liège: Ordina Editions, 1982 (For the International Union for the Scientific Study of Population).

U.S. Department of Health and Human Services Task Force on Health Risk Assessment: *Determining Risks to Health—Federal Policy and Practice.* Dover, MA: Auburn House, 1986.

U.S. House of Representatives: *A Discursive Dictionary of Health Care.* Washington DC: US Government Printing Office, 1976.

Webster's Third New International Dictionary, Unabridged. Springfield, MA: Merriam, 1971.

Weed LL: *Medical Records, Medical Education and Patient Care.* Cleveland: Case Western Reserve University Press, 1969.

White KL, Henderson M (Eds): *Epidemiology as a Fundamental Science.* New York: Oxford University Press, 1976.

Wilson C: *The Dictionary of Demography* (Translation from the French of Roland Pressat). Oxford: Blackwell, 1985.

World Bank: *A Glossary of Population Terminology.* Washington: World Bank, 1985.

World Organization of National Colleges, Academies (WONCA) of Family Practice: *International Classification of Health Problems in Primary Care,* 3rd ed. Oxford: Oxford University Press. In Press, 1987.